Airtight Pulmonary Function Tests

Coaching Tips from Real Life Experiences

Rosemary McWilliams,
BAS, RRT, CPFT

All scripture quotations, unless otherwise indicated, are taken from the Amplified Bible, Copyright © 1954, 1958, 1962, 1964, 1965, 1987 by The Lockman Foundation. Used by permission.

ISBN-13: 978-1500191856

Library of Congress: 2011946301

Rosemary (R.K.) McWilliams, BAS, RRT, CPFT

Author Website: http://rkmcwilliams.com

Email: rk@rkmcwilliams.com

Gold Writer Publishing

Contents

To the One who gave me breath

and sustains me.

To my husband, my

strongest encourager.

To my family who loves me just as I am.

To my parents who would have

been very proud.

And to my friend, Kelly, who

just wanted her name in a book.

Preface

The sixteen-year-old came bouncing into the office with her mother, who had worry written on her face. The teen held the results of a pulmonary function test (PFT) in her hand and was told she probably had asthma, or did she? That was why she was at the pulmonologist's office—to determine if that was truly the case.

I looked at the test and thought, "Ugh, this is one of the worst tests I've ever seen." The age was wrong, the height was a whopping five inches off, and the report stated that the patient could not produce acceptable results. The forced vital capacity (FVC) test was abnormal at 69 percent, and she only blew out for two seconds instead of six. "Why?" I wondered. She looked young, bright, and healthy. Does she have a learning disorder preventing her from doing the simple spirometry test? Her mother said they made her blow out at least ten times but always told her she was not doing it correctly!

I measured her height and weight and then started with the forced vital capacity test. I explained it to her, using the coaching skills I've learned over 34 years of pulmonary function testing, and she performed it accurately and perfectly. She did a complete test with lung volumes, lung diffusion, and body plethysmography without difficulty. What was the difference this time? Accurate information and good coaching skills.

This is an example of the great need in our field to ramp up our skills, whether it is just a simple spirometry test, or complete pulmonary function testing done in a lab. Therefore, I am sharing some secrets I've learned over the years.

Introduction

This book is for everyone who has done, is doing, or will be doing pulmonary function testing in a hospital, school, research lab, physician's office, or corporate setting. It will open your eyes to the various people groups you will be testing. Whether you are giving an annual employee spirometry test, a pre-op test, a disability test, or monitoring a COPD patient, you will learn helpful hints and tips. You will recognize common errors in coaching and see how to correct them.

This is information you will not find in your regular textbooks, but can be used to enhance your knowledge of pulmonary function testing. Whether you are new to the field, or it has been your lifelong career, you will find *Airtight Pulmonary Function Tests* a refreshing read filled with "real life" experiences and helpful tips.

I encourage you to test this knowledge and prove it to yourself and your clients. Not only will you benefit from this material, but your patients/clients will be happier and more cooperative. As you begin to understand the essentials of coaching techniques, a new understanding of your clients develops, resulting in better cooperation and PFT results. It is presented to encourage you in your work and practice as a pulmonary function technologist. Have fun!

Chapter 1

A PFT IS TO THE LUNGS AS AN EKG AS TO THE HEART

Pulmonary function tests determine how well the lungs are functioning. Similarly, an EKG tells how well the heart is beating. This is quite basic. However, when tests are done poorly, the information is unusable and may lead to misdiagnosis. Therefore, good coaching skills are essential for pulmonary function test accuracy.

PFT results help identify various lung diseases and determine severity. It may be just one test or many tests, depending on the purpose. For example, if a firefighter or an asbestos worker needs an annual PFT, a simple spirometry test is adequate to determine the forced vital capacity (FVC) and the forced expiratory volume in the 1st second of time (FEV1). But, a person with chronic obstructive pulmonary disease (COPD) may require additional tests, such as lung volumes and lung diffusion.

There are various reasons for PFTs, such as pre-operative testing, diagnosis of lung diseases, monitoring changes in a known lung disease, to determine effectiveness of medications, and for disability evaluation. Results of a PFT may or may not allow a young adult into the military due to asthma. Or they may alert an anesthesiologist to a high-risk patient. A person's health care plan and medications may change based on the results of a PFT. PFTs are used to monitor long-term drug effects from Amiodarone, an antiarrythmic heart medication, and Methotrexate, used to relieve rheumatoid arthritis. *PFTs have the ability to alter a person's life course forever.* Therefore, they must be taken seriously, as we strive to get the most accurate results possible.

PFTs require cooperation between the technologist administering the test and the person taking the test. The tests are effort-dependent and each test must be performed in a certain manner. The American Thoracic Society (ATS) and European Respiratory Society (ERS) have developed guidelines for obtaining acceptable test results in an effort to standardize testing procedures. (See http://www.thoracic.org/statements/).

Various parameters, such as height, weight, race, and machine calibration can affect the results of a test. Information is entered into the pulmonary function machine, so the "predicted normals" for a patient can be pulled up and compared to the patient's actual effort. The computer then calculates a percentage of predicted results, which can indicate obstruction and/or restriction in the lungs and other alterations in values.

Let's Get Better At This

All too often, patients come into a pulmonary lab for retesting because of abnormal PFTs. But many times we find, after retesting that the patient's lung functions were not abnormal; there were just inaccuracies in patient information and test performance. For example, these findings included:

1. A spirometry test showed a 56-year-old female to have an abnormal forced vital capacity (FVC) of 78 percent and a forced expiratory volume in the 1st second (FEV1) of 72 percent. Examination of the test revealed an incorrect patient height (four inches taller than she actually was) and the machine had not been calibrated for over a month. Also, the report clearly indicated that ATS guidelines were not met because the efforts were not acceptable and repeatable, even though the warnings were printed to coach the patient to "blow out longer" and "blast out faster." After retesting in our lab with good coaching and in full compliance with

ATS standards, the patient's FVC was actually supra-normal at 105 percent of predicted results.

2. A lung diffusion test with a value of zero but reported as an accurate test.

3. A flattened forced vital capacity (FVC) graph on an otherwise healthy teenager, which reflected poor effort and coaching. Read more about the Teen Phenomenon in Chapter Five.

4. And, our real life example in the preface of our sixteen-year-old who thought she may have asthma.

These are just a few of the many examples which illustrate the need for better coaching techniques, attention to accuracy of patient information, and review of the test results. As we become more skillful at PFTs, we can give our patients quality care. Remember:

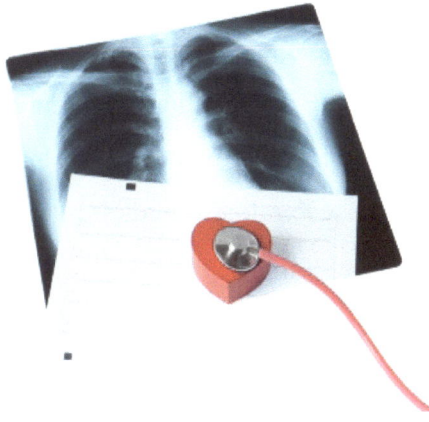

A PFT is to the Lungs as an EKG is to the Heart!

I Dread This Test!

A gentleman came into the office for a PFT. He looked at the machine and immediately said, "Oh, I dread this test." It is always saddening to hear comments like that, and, unfortunately, I used to hear them a lot! I asked him why he felt that way and he said the man made him blow so long, "I just couldn't stand it." Even though he had the test done many years ago, it still haunted him. I said I would try to make this a much better experience for him. When he was done, he said, "Oh, that wasn't so bad." I was successful in changing his mind about PF testing, which was one of my goals. And, most importantly, the tests were accurate and of good repeatable quality per American Thoracic Society standards.

(Note: The ATS is a non-profit organization of more than 15,000 physicians, scientists, and other allied, healthcare professionals from around the world who establish standards of care for respiratory disorders, pediatric asthma, sleep disorders, pulmonary function testing, infectious diseases, thoracic surgery, critical care and more. The ERS is an international medical organization of more than 10,000 members, formed to share knowledge, improve education, and establish standards in the field of respiratory medicine. See http://dev.ersnet.org/10-overview.htm.)

Uno Mas

One more anecdote. Another gentleman came in for a test, but he did not mention any negative experiences with previous PFTs. He was very pleasant and his PFT efforts were excellent. Later on, the office manager said to me, "Mr. R. said his previous PFT experiences were something he would rather forget, but you made it a pleasant experience and he is actually looking forward to his next PF test!" As we improve our coaching skills, we will have happier patients and get better results.

Quality PFTs

So, why are some PFT experiences horrible and other not? PFTs have been given a bad name and I believe this mindset can be turned around greatly by learning new coaching techniques. I want to show the technologist that you can get quality tests from patients without "torturing" them into submission. Perhaps only a few changes in your coaching techniques will get desired effects. We can't expect 100 percent success, but we can expect:

1. Less complaints from patients/clients.

2. Writing "patient unable to perform tests" less often.

3. A less stressful job (yours).

4. Quality tests that fulfill ATS/ERS requirements.

5. A happier employer (physician, Medical Director or corporation).

6. Properly done PFTs for disability determination.

7. Properly done PFTs for pre-op surgery.

8. Properly done PFTs for military entrance.

9. Proper and consistently done PFTs for research.

10. Consistency in annual employee spirometries.

11. Consistency between co-worker coaching and testing techniques.

12. Credibility for yourself and the tests you perform.

Even though this is a specialized field, there are people with a wide variety of backgrounds administering PFTs. These include lay people, office staff members, nurses, registered respiratory therapists (RRT), physicians or other medical personnel. Some have little training; some have been trained by the PF machine manufacturers; some have read a manual; and others have been certified by the National Board for Respiratory Care (NBRC) as registered pulmonary function technologists (RPFT) and certified pulmonary function technologists (CPFT).

The United States OSHA regulations require the tester to have a minimum 16 hours of training approved by the National Institute for Occupational Safety and Health (NIOSH) for everyone, except physicians, who perform PFTs. They have approximately 29 testing sites throughout the country. You can also download a spirometry instruction manual and a great chart entitled, "Get Valid Spirometry Results EVERY Time." (See http://www.cdc.gov/niosh/docs/2011-135/pdfs/2011-135.pdf). This chart shows how to correct test errors, and graphically shows how to identify leaks, glottis closures, or other common problems. For more information, see http://www.cdc.gov/niosh/topics/spirometry/training.html.

Another well-respected organization, Global Initiative for Chronic Obstructive Lung Disease (GOLD) has a spirometry guide you may download by going to http://www.goldcopd.org/.

The current ATS/ERS recommendation is two years of college education and familiarization with the equipment, techniques, calibrations, and quality controls. They also recommend spirometer refresher training. However, for the overall majority, there are no written requirements for training for those who administer PFTs. Therefore, there is a wide variety of skills in this field.

This lack of standardization has caused a difference of opinion between these agencies and medical professionals, many of whom believe only trained, qualified professionals should administer PFTs. This on-going debate has not produced guidelines as of yet, which makes the information provided in this book even more vital.

In an effort toward global standardization, the ATS/ERS Task Force has written "Standardisation of Spirometry," "Standardisation of Lung Volume Measurement," "CO Diffusing Capacity Standardisation" and more. These standards are necessary for consistency in PFT machines, calibration, testing procedures, and result selection. They can be found online at the American Thoracic Society website: http://www.thoracic.org/statements/ . I highly encourage you to read the standards.

Over twenty-eight years ago, a pulmonologist told me, "If the patient is not more short of breath after the test, you haven't done your job." True, many people with severe COPD, emphysema, and other obstructive lung diseases may get very short of breath during the testing. However, there are ways to help them through the testing so it is not such a difficult and miserable experience, and without sacrificing good, quality results. It is better not to cut corners, muddle through, or be in too much of a hurry when it comes to PFTs. Take the time to care.

Chapter 2

A FRESH APPROACH

This is not a technical manual but a fresh, new look at the art of pulmonary function testing. This new approach looks more closely at the people taking the tests, their lung disease and personality traits and how to coach them into getting acceptable test results. When we apply a little psychology to our coaching methods and dialogue, we have much greater success in obtaining quality results on the majority of people.

People Groups

Even though people are individuals, they are alike in many ways. This is especially true when it comes to disease groups. Throughout the years, I have observed various "people groups" who seem to fall into categories. I will define some of the most common types you will encounter and then explain how to coach the patient to get the best results for each individual people group. This is a virtually untouched area of pulmonary function testing. Often, PF technicians are taught to do tests on healthy, cooperative co-workers or supervisors; so, when a patient with severe COPD comes in for a test, suddenly the skills they learned don't seem to apply. Usually, that patient cannot be coached as if he or she has "*normal*" lungs.

Not all respiratory therapy schools have trained pulmonary function instructors, so they may have to rely on hospital staff or others to teach students. When your employer purchases a PFT machine, they often include a training package for the therapist who will be giving the tests. Some of the best education I received was from these corporations. There are excellent manuals written generically by manufacturers of pulmonary function machines, which offer instructions on how to coach the patient/client.

This text covers traditional PF tests, not High-End Impulse Oscillometry (IOS) which is used to determine respiratory impedance of the lung-thorax system.

Five Universal PFT Laws

Since 1979, I have done pulmonary function testing at various organizations across four different states. As I studied people everywhere, I learned what to do, what not to do, what words to say, and what attitude works best. As a result, I have learned tricks, tips, techniques, and how to get a good pulmonary function test from even the most difficult of patients. After all, that is the goal. The physician who ordered the test is expecting quality results done according to ATS/ ERS standards and the five universal PFT laws will help you achieve this goal.

Practically anyone can learn how to coach people into performing pulmonary function testing, but can you get a high percentage of them to perform the tests properly for acceptable results? Here are some universal laws that I have discovered to aid the technologist in PF coaching methods. These laws apply for a simple spirometry test, or a complete PFT with lung volumes, lung diffusion (DLCO), or more.

The five universal PFT laws will help the pulmonary function technologistlearn the quickest, easiest ways to achieve success in getting quality tests. You will greatly reduce the number of patients who previously would have fallen into the "unable to perform testing" category. I call them the Mac Laws:

Mac Law 1: Please Don't Shout—Communicate

Mac Law 2: Less Info, Better Results

Mac Law 3: I Relax, You Relax, We All Relax

Mac Law 4: Encourage Now, Then and Again

Mac Law 5: My Attitude Is Everything

These laws are mentioned here to familiarize you with the general concepts, but they will be defined and examined more closely in subsequent chapters. You will also see how the laws work together, shown by the examples in this book.

Although it may take an average employee many months to learn a job, the skills to obtain quality pulmonary function tests may take years to learn. Hopefully, the information presented here, will give you insight into shortening the learning process. These laws do not, in any way, violate the ATS/ERS standards for pulmonary function testing, nor are they intended to replace, duplicate, or alter them.

Real Life Experience

Reality. It's the fad of the decade, dominating television and entertainment with real people (versus actors) looking for money, success and happiness. Here you'll find real life experiences which illustrate and explain the Mac Laws and how they were developed. Some experiences are humorous, but, whether entertaining or not, all serve to teach technologists excellent coaching skills in administering pulmonary function tests.

A Readable Book

I purposely made this book more attractive by keeping it just the right length; not too short and not too long (and boring). The average length of time people will wait for a website to pull up is usually 10-20 seconds and then they move on. Some say people will only wait four seconds. So, what has that to do with this book? The basic principle is that people are just BUSY. Does every college student read every word in every book for every course? It would be nice, but it just isn't reality. Therefore, if you can make a book short, down to basics, interesting, and add a touch of humor, it will have a much higher chance of being fully read and understood. That is my goal.

Chapter 3

THE MAC LAWS

Mac Law 1: Please Don't Shout-Communicate

Reality: I rolled the spirometer into the room, to meet my next patient. He was 6'4" tall and weighed 320 pounds. I coached him shouting, "BLOW, BLOW, BLOW!" He stopped, looked at me with tears in his eyes and whimpered, "Please don't shout!"

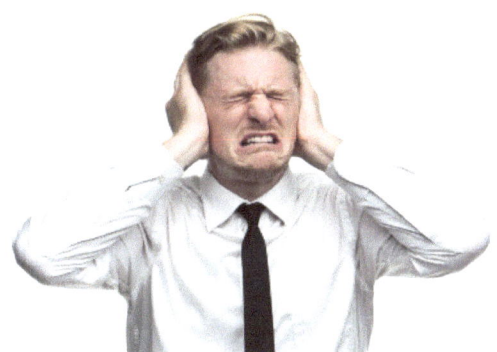

Please Don't Shout!

It was quite unexpected to realize that his sensitivity was at odds with his stature. I try to learn something from everyone I meet, and this gentle giant awakened me to a better approach in coaching pulmonary function tests. We are taught to be enthusiastic when coaching people to get good quality PFTs. However, sometimes we interpret that eagerness to mean being loud and aggressive. This illustration proves that this type of coaching does not work on all people. People are not all the same, yet we attempt to do PFTs the same way to all people. This incident birthed

Mac Law 1: Please Don't Shout—Communicate, which is the first of five universal laws for pulmonary function testing.

When doing a spirometry test, it is not necessary to shout at the client when encouraging him or her to blow, blow, blow. There are people who respond poorly when yelled at, but we still need to get good PFT results. To this end, we are taught to be enthusiastic in coaching with our words and body language. We can do that very effectively when we first find the correct volume and tone of voice and, then, stress certain words during the coaching. It also doesn't hurt to advise the patient/client that you may have to raise your voice, but not to take it personally, as it is just the nature of the test.

The key is communication. Learn to be a great communicator and your "simple" spirometry just might turn out to be simple.

Reality: A client was getting a pulmonary function test done and after the first few tests she finally said to the technician, "Maybe I can't breathe, but I'm not deaf!"

Reality: One day, an ICU nurse grumbled that some of the PF technicians shouted so loudly when doing bedside spirometries that it disturbed the other patients in the unit. It is not good for ICU patients to be irritated!

Reality: The PF technician yelled, "BLOW," and everyone in the room jumped.

Reality: A technician used a moderate tone and volume while coaching a patient through PFTs, yet had great success in obtaining quality tests.

Reality: A friend was having his annual spirometry at his workplace. I asked how it went and he said the nurse told him to put the mouthpiece in his mouth and blow as hard as he could for as long as he could. However, she did not coach him DURING the test and it took many repetitions to obtain acceptable results. This is an example of no volume being just as bad as too much volume!

So, what is the correct volume or loudness of voice? Learn to use a volume that is moderate and put the emphasis on the first word, such as BLOW or BLAST; then taper off. Listen to the patients and if they object to your volume, adjust it accordingly. Some people are hard of hearing so, of course, you may have to talk louder to them.

Besides volume, our voices have pitch and tone. Pitch is the degree of highness or lowness in a sound or tone, determined by the rate of vibrations producing it; while tone is the use of pitch or pitch changes.

Tone is the character of a sound. It is the shrillness and depth of a sound. For example, several instruments playing the same note are in the same pitch but the depth of tone is what distinguishes one instrument from another. Therefore, a trumpet sounds different from a clarinet. The technician, who startled everyone in the room, had difficulty with both loudness and tone.

It is the tone that sets the mood because it generates emotions, not logic—as you converse with someone. Therefore, it is important to consider the emotions that you are presenting from the tone of your voice. Are they proper emotions? When giving PFTs, it is so true that, what we say is important, but how we say it may be even more important. After all, what makes a cheerful voice different from an angry voice? Or, a thankful voice different from a frustrated voice? It's the loudness, pitch, and especially tone.

What character (tone) does your voice display when giving PFTs? Listen to yourself as you coach the patient. Be deliberate and honest about your self-evaluation.

Because our voices are different, we each must find our perfect sound for coaching the individual to obtain the best results. Once you find that optimum sound, stick with it and it will work for the majority of patients.

Be patient with yourself and ask your clients how you are doing. Most people are very willing to help, especially when they are on the receiving end. You can also ask your supervisor and co-workers for a critique of your voice qualities. It really doesn't take long to find your range, but you will have better success if you start out at a moderate volume and tone, then adjust as needed from there. If you work alone, try recording yourself—you may be surprised.

However, if you are not getting the results you need from your patient, such as a quick, sharp blast of air on the first second of the forced vital capacity (FVC) test, then you will know to increase your volume a notch. Also, learn to be more expressive in your body language. When asking a patient to take in a deep breath, wave your arm and hand upwards. When you say, "BLAST it out," bring your arm down quickly. It is very effective to use visuals. Enthusiastically use facial expressions, arms, hands and demonstration to get your point across.

For example: You have a client in your office that just can't seem to follow your expert coaching and instructions. Nothing you try seems to work. Let's look at improving your body language. Just a few simple changes may improve the results. During a deep inspiration maneuver, raise your arm high, indicating a deep breath in. Then, quickly drop it when you say, "BLOW." Just make sure you are not sitting too close to the patient when you do arm movements, so as not to startle and distract him or her.

During a maximum voluntary ventilation (MVV) test, demonstrate with your own breathing and by moving your hand up and down in rhythm. Hand signals also work very well for the vital capacity (VC) maneuver and the body plethysmography panting maneuver. Such gestures are a must for patients who are hard of hearing. You can point up when asking for a deep breath and down for exhalation.

While performing the PF tests, be sure your client can see your face. Move your equipment if necessary and speak clearly.

You can even use facial expressions to get your client to obtain a better seal on the mouthpiece. Say, "Put your lips forward, like you are kissing." Then, show the client. Don't laugh, it works! Most people will understand immediately.

Mac Law 2: Less Info, Better Results

This law will make your job so much easier! For years, I coached patients by telling them they should blow out for at least six seconds for the forced vital capacity (FVC) test or that they would hold their breaths for ten seconds on the lung diffusion (DLCO) test. Never again. When you throw out numbers like that, most people will respond, "If I can," or, "I don't think I can do that." I learned that less information means better results. Just keep your coaching simple.

Reality: After a long, drawn-out explanation, the patient said to me, "Now I start out how? I do what?"

Reality: After telling the patient that he should hold his breath for ten seconds, he said, "Well, I'll try, but I don't think I can hold it that long!"

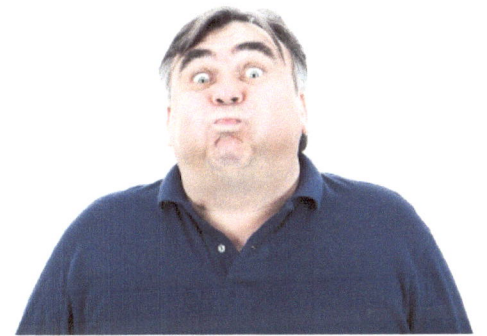

Hold It, Hold It, Hold It!

Reality: After telling the patient he would be blowing out a minimum of six seconds, he said, "Six seconds, are you trying to kill me?"

Many people with COPD, asthma, restrictive lung disease (RLD), and other breathing problems know they are limited in their breathing, so they do not think they can do the tests properly. Therefore, encourage them to understand that the machine will only be measuring what they *can* do.

It is better to present your information at a high school level or an educational level lower than you would normally speak about the subject you know so well. This strategy is not to insult their intelligence, but rather keeps it clear of technical jargon. It is not necessary to convey everything you know about the testing to your client. You will see that this law works for many of the groups, especially the "I Can't Character."

For example, it is better to not sound like a textbook when you are coaching someone. Don't say, "You will take approximately four tidal breaths, then inhale maximally to your inspiratory capacity, and then blow out to RV." Those medicals terms and acronyms don't mean anything to the patient.

Keep your instructions to a minimum in order that the patient does not get confused. Some patients will attempt to try to remember your directions, so let them know right away that they don't have to memorize anything, because you'll be coaching them through each step (see Chapter Four, Coaching Scripts).

If you have a patient who just does not seem to understand, try changing your words. Find better explanations until you get the results you need.

Mac Law 3: I Relax, You Relax, We All Relax

"Calmness is power." James Allen

The above statement deserves to be a Law. Why? Because a great number of people with breathing difficulties experience panic, fear, tenseness, nervousness and anxiety in varying degrees. It is so important for the technologist to create a stress-free, relaxed environment. Often, those who struggle with breathing will be anxious before they get to the pulmonary lab. Numerous patients talk about their "panicky" feeling. This concern is very real and should not be ignored. It is important for both the technologist and the client to be as relaxed as possible. Also, your own nervousness can be sensed, so learn to reduce it to a minimum.

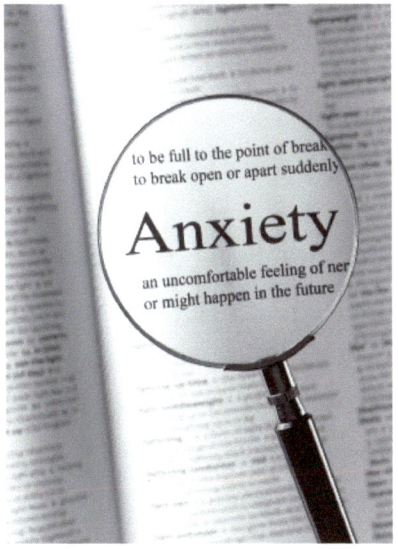

Reality: An individual with severe COPD mentioned that he sleeps with a fan blowing on him, even if the temperature outside is 20 below zero. He says that it makes him feel better, especially when he gets that "panicky" feeling and can't breathe. Before we started the PFT, he said he didn't think he was breathing well enough to do the tests. But, he was just anxious. After relaxing, he was able to do a pre and post spirometry, body plethysmograph (body box), and lung diffusion (DLCO). He actually did better than he thought he would.

Reality: A young lady came in for a pulmonary function test and was performing all the tests just fine, with normal values. Then, we started the nitrogen washout test for lung volumes. After breathing normally for a couple of minutes, she suddenly panicked and came off the machine gasping, "I can't breathe!" So, what happened? She was doing fine until then. Nothing had changed with the test or the machine. She simply talked herself into a panic. Her mind was allowed to think "too much."

Reality: Occasionally technicians may become nervous and overly excited when administering the DLCO test. Their elevated voices also elevate the stress level in the room.

There is a lot you can do to create a relaxed atmosphere in your lab or office. Consider playing soft, relaxing music in the background. A water feature sits on my desk, which is relaxing in sight and sound. Next to it, is a vase filled with artificial, hanging flowers that move gently in the breeze of the air conditioner.

Conversation can be relaxing too. Strike up a conversation by finding common ground. The picture of my Shih Tzu, Critter, on the computer screen, often becomes the topic of conversation, since so many of my patients have little lap dogs or cats.

Then there is common courtesy, which activates a relaxed atmosphere. It is polite and advantageous to use the patient's name and use it often. People like to hear their names. Since I have lived in Texas, I got used to saying, "Sir" and "Ma'am." Respect goes a long way. And don't forget to introduce yourself. Get in the habit, as soon as you meet your client, to tell him or her, your name and job title. One of my pet peeves is going to a medical facility, whether it be the ophthalmologist or an emergency department, and people rush in and out without any explanation of who they are and what they are there to do.

Offer tissues and a drink of water. Offer a good, clean joke to get your client laughing and relaxed. If your client wears oxygen, offer to put the patient on an oxygen concentrator to conserve his or her portable tank. Consider your client's needs.

Also, be careful to keep your hands to yourself, as many people do not like to be touched. Occasionally, a situation will arise when it is better for a man to administer a test to a man or a woman to a woman, or to keep the door open during the test.

Please do not wear perfumes, use scented sprays, or scented hand wash. Scents can aggravate the airways for many people.

Reality: An elderly lady with COPD came in for an annual PFT but wears so much talc that *my* airways react instantly. I'm the one who ends up needing a breathing treatment!

Now, a quick review. Reduce stress by using Mac Law 1 (Please Don't Shout) and coach with a calm voice. Use Mac Law 2 (Less Info, Better Results) so as not to overload your clients with unnecessary information that could only stress them out more. Practice Mac Law 3 (I Relax, You Relax, We All Relax). Relaxing is not just for the client, but also those giving the test. If you are nervous, it shows. To overcome your own nervousness, act confidently, learn as much as you can about doing your job effectively (by reading this book), read the ATS/ERS standards, and take the CPFT and RPFT tests. Building your education can build your confidence. Become the expert in your area. Also, belong to and support your local respiratory associations and American Association for Respiratory Care. Building your resume builds confidence. Begin by believing in yourself!

The Bartender Syndrome

So often, in the PF lab, I feel like a bartender listening to the problems of the world. I have heard personal, intimate details of things that only a professional counselor should hear. I have listened to stories of injustices from the government, healthcare system and political groups.

Family fights and feuds are a big topic. And, oh, that neighbor down the block. "He lets his dog do his business in my yard!" And, on and on...the Complaint Department is open!

So, how can Mac Law 3 (I Relax, Your Relax, We All Relax) apply to the bartender syndrome? Listen to the patients. Yes, listen. Let them pour out their concerns. Conversation is an important step to relaxation. If they trust you enough with personal information, the defenses are down and ears open to your instructions. You may get a better PFT. Due to time constraints, however, you may need to control the conversation, by leading your client into the next test, which is easy to do.

People are interesting and so are their stories and experiences. Some really do need someone with whom to talk. It doesn't hurt to be that someone for the short amount of time you spend with them.

However, it is not all complaints. I have laughed with, prayed with, had my heart touched by, encouraged by, learned from, received social contacts from, and been inspired by many clients.

Mac Law 4: Encourage Now, Then, and Again

"A happy heart is good medicine and a cheerful mind works healing."
Proverbs 17:22

Encouragement comes in many forms. It is the positive, encouraging words you may say, facial expressions and body language you use, and the smile you present. Even an expression of compassion can reflect encouragement towards the patient.

Words of Encouragement

I spend a great deal of time encouraging clients. They need to hear, "good effort," "good job," or "you're doing great." Everyone loves words of encouragement. Just make it clear that you are evaluating their performance not the test results.

Another method of encouragement is giving out positive statements that lessen anxiety, such as: "Most tests take less than a minute to do." And "I will explain each test before you do it, but you don't have to memorize the directions (smile) because I'll coach you through it." When people hear positives, they do much better on the tests.

My coaching scripts have changed to "asking," not "telling" clients what to do. For example: I'll *ask* you to take in a deep breath and then to blow it out hard and fast. One simple word can stimulate cooperation in your client, especially in the Controller (See Chapter Five.)

Another substitute is to use the word "say." For example: "I will *say* take in a deep breath and then to blow it out hard and fast."

Mac Law 4 (Encourage Now, Then and Again) works very well with the lung volume tests, whether done by nitrogen washout, helium dilution, or body plethysmography. Talk almost continually to your patients, encouraging and praising their efforts. As they listen to your voice, they will concentrate on your words, not on their breathing or how they are "feeling." For example, say:

> *You are doing fine. Just keep breathing as you are.*

> *We are getting there.*

> *You are doing very well; just keep breathing normally.*

Using an abundance of encouraging words helps your clients relax, and relaxation cause better PFTs.

Smile

"A smile is the beginning of peace." Mother Teresa

Smiles are so amazingly powerful and influencing. Look at all they do:

- Create a welcoming atmosphere.

- Help your client to relax.

- Help you to relax.

- Calm anxious patients by reducing stress and insecurity over test performance.

- Make you attractive and approachable.

- Initiate a positive response. People smile back!

- Tell people they are accepted.

- Instantly change attitudes and grumpy old men to more pleasant ones.

- Send out feel-good endorphins, natural pain relievers and serotonin to your body with similar effects as morphine, without the hallucinations!

- Measurably reduce blood pressure.

- Boost the immune system by reducing the cortisol hormone.

- Improve mental health.

Try to think of some more benefits to smiling. There are many. A smile is a gift everyone has been given, which should be given back to others. Think of it as another form of therapy that you can give. It costs you nothing and benefits everyone.

Many people have breathing problems, and the focus of their daily living is getting the next breath. Some days, this difficulty can discourage even the happiest of extroverts. So, we need to be compassionate and make their smiles for them. Even if they crack a little smile, things can improve. The endorphins will kick in and then emotional and physical healing can begin.

Body Language

Use encouraging body signals, such as:

- When appropriate, shake hands with your client when you meet.

- During conversation lean toward your client slightly, indicating you are listening.

- Hold your gaze as you converse, slowly nodding to encourage him/her to continue.

- Repeat your client's words or phrases to affirm what he/she is saying.

Mac Law 5: My Attitude is Everything

"What is the hardest thing in life to face? Yourself." Rosemary McWilliams

You can make the pulmonary function testing the best possible experience for the patient and yourself—or the worst—just by your attitude. Therefore, let's make it the best.

First, you must honestly examine your own demeanor. We can be blind to our own ways, but I invite you to begin looking at yourself; your words, your tone, facial expressions, behavior, and general attitude. Have the courage to ask for help from co-workers. Ask your supervisor how you are doing. Doing this exercise has an added advantage because, when your evaluation is due, you may get a better one, since you will already have had time to work on your areas of improvement.

We know that the first impression is important. People notice your face, smile, clothes, stature, walk, words, and tone of voice—all within a few minutes. If you look angry, sad, or negative, their response to you will reflect what they encounter. Be approachable. When you wear a smile, they see friendliness. Often, your demeanor even overrides the clothes you are wearing. But don't let that stop you from dressing professionally.

A perceptive person can read your body language. It reveals if you are frustrated, pressed for time, or having a bad day. Be aware of the mood you display—and give your client top priority by serving him first. Then, deal with your mood later.

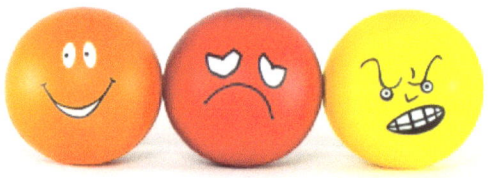

My Attitude is Everything

Confidence

"Confidence is the most attractive coat I can wear." Rosemary McWilliams

To exhibit confidence, walk with your head level and use good eye contact. People tend to feel comfortable and secure when confronted with a confident person. Let your demeanor exude calm confidence. If you don't feel that way, practice or pretend that you do; and, eventually, it will become a habit and, hopefully, a part of who you are.

Think about it, would you mimic someone who is not confident? No, we mimic and learn from successful people.

Patience

I know, sometimes you will get the most frustrating people in the lab that will push your patience to the limit. Remember, "calmness is power." Also, have empathy for the patient. Besides breathing problems, you never know what else a person is experiencing. An angry person may be upset with his/her spouse, daughter, health condition or financial situation and you may be the target for the moment, but it is only for a moment.

Reality: I went to get my next PFT patient from the hospital waiting room. Immediately, he said, "Well it's about time!" Actually, he was an hour early. I explained that I can test only one patient at a time and the machine was busy. He didn't want to hear any explanation. He continued on and on, in anger, which was beginning to annoy me. I told him that I was going to get another therapist to do his test, since I seemed to aggravate him. It was then that he calmed down and apologized. He said he was scheduled for major surgery in the morning and was afraid he would not make it off the table. He was angry about it and took his frustrations out on me.

This man was very frightened and I just happened to be the nearest target for his emotions. I was going to switch with my co-worker, who could get along with a raging bull and I knew that she could calm him down. If you have the luxury of tag teaming, do it!

Reality: A lady came into the lab and said she really didn't like these tests. When questioned why, she explained that the last technician got frustrated with her when she did not do the test correctly, which made her even more nervous. I said, "I will try to make this a much better experience for you." After the testing, she thanked me for being so patient, and for not putting pressure on her. She complimented me on having a calm voice, which helped her performance anxiety. Keep all frustration in check. It never helps the situation.

Then, there is the client who just doesn't seem to follow directions properly. You've pre-coached, coached, demonstrated and done the maximum attempts, but he or she simply does not understand. This is your challenge. You are dealing with someone who has the power to transform you through chiseling and sculpting your patience—a transformer, seeking to get on your last nerve. Will you be transformed and pass the test?

I've failed many of those tests, but I am not a failure. A failure is one who doesn't try again. Each success is a step toward mastery. Like climbing stairs, you keep advancing with each encounter with a transformer. If you don't have patience, you will learn it through the people with whom you come in contact. Just let it happen. Your tests and your life will be better for it.

Use a Soothing Voice

Reality: A patient told me that my voice is very soothing as I coached her through the PFTs and she appreciated that, saying, "It helps me to relax and do better."

I remember hearing my voice for the first time in elementary school. The teacher hauled out one of those reel-to-reel tape recorders and put it on her desk. One by one, we filed up there to say a sentence into the recorder. She thought it would be good for us to become familiar with our own voice. I thought I was going to die. My shyness overwhelmed me and I talked in a whisper. When I heard my voice, I did not like it and put my head down on the desk. If only I could have seen into the future, that one day I would actually sing at my brother's wedding!

Through the years, I learned to speak. I used to blurt out whatever was on my mind, but now I carefully choose words to create the right atmosphere. Be courteous; speak slowly and steadily. Learn to control your voice with composure. Using words seasoned with grace is always the right choice.

Chapter 4

COACHING SCRIPTS

"Lucy, you got some 'splainin' to do!" Desi Arnaz

Here are some universal coaching scripts that work well for most of the people, most of the time. However, because of the wide variety of pulmonary function machines in use today, these coaching scripts are offered as a guide.

In this text, *pre-test coaching* refers to the words (script) you speak to the client *before* he/she takes the test. This gives your client an idea of what to expect. *Coaching* refers to the words you speak to the client *as* he/she is taking the test on the pulmonary function machine.

Before testing, prepare the patient by a brief explanation of the test procedure.

- *I will put a filter and mouthpiece on the machine through which you will be breathing for all the tests.*

- *You will also wear nose clips so the machine can measure all the air that you breathe through your mouth.*

- *You'll be doing several different tests that will tell us a lot about the condition of your lungs.*

- *I'll explain each test before you do it, to give you an idea of what to expect.*

- *But you don't have to memorize anything because I will coach you through each test, as you are doing it.* (Smile)

- *Each test does not take long to do—usually less than a minute—but we have to get several efforts of each test for accuracy.*

This script is simple and direct, with no confusion. Immediately, your patient knows that all he or she needs to do is to listen and follow your coaching.

Spirometry Coaching: The "Blow, Blow, Blow" Test

Spirometry is simply a test done on a spirometer machine, which measures volumes of air being inhaled and exhaled over time.

This is the basic test used for pre-employment physicals, annual physicals, cystic fibrosis checkups, disability testing and military entrance testing. Sometimes, it is called an FVC (forced vital capacity), or an FVL (flow volume loop) or spirometry. Basically, an FVL is an FVC with a deep and maximal inspiration added to the end.

It is a quick way to identify obstruction in the lungs. Or, it may indicate restriction and the need for further studies, such as lung volumes. A quick look at the FVC, FEV1 and the FVC/FEV1% gives us a lot of information. Also, the FEF25-75% on a well-done test may reflect the condition of the small airways. Prepare the patient for a FVL with a quick explanation:

- *On this test, you will begin by breathing normally on the mouthpiece.*

- *Then, I will ask you to take in a deep breath—all the way in.*

- *Next, I'll say to BLAST it out as hard and fast as you can and to keep pushing it out*

- *UNTIL I say to take in another deep breath.*

- *You will empty way, way out.*

- *You may empty out before I say to take in another deep breath; and, if you do, don't take in a breath.*

- *Instead, continue to try pushing it out or even hold it there if you have to.*

- *But don't take in a breath until I ask you to do so.*

Alternate Script: (This works well too!)

- *You'll be on the mouthpiece, with the nose clips on, breathing normally.*

- *Then, I'll ask you to take in a deep breath—all the way in.*

- *Then, I'll say to BLAST it out hard and fast.*

- *You will blow it out as HARD as you can for as LONG as you can, or maybe a little longer!* (Smile)

- *You'll be very empty; and then, at the end, I'll ask you to take in another quick, deep breath.*

At this point, you will get a spirometry attempt from the patient. (Coach the patient during the test, using this as a guide.)

- *Breathe normally.*

- (at end of expiration) *Now, take in a deep breath, all the way.* (raising your arm up high)

- *Now BLAST it out.* (Drop arm down quickly.) *Keep blowing; keep blowing; let it out all the way; keep blowing . . . almost there.*

- (Get a minimum of six seconds expiration for adults, three seconds for children.)

- *OK, now take in a fast, deep breath.*

- *Great effort. Relax and take the mouthpiece out of your mouth.*

- *When you feel ready, we'll get another one.*

Evaluate the patient's effort and the graph. You will immediately be able to tell:

1. If it was a good or poor effort.

2. If the blast out was hard enough.

3. If the blast was long enough.

4. If there is lung restriction (completely or near empty after just a few seconds of a forceful exhalation).

5. If there is lung obstruction (takes forever to empty out).

If the blast was not hard enough, you may say:

- *That was good for the first attempt.*

- *What we can do to make that better is this:*

- *The first second, when you start to blow, you will blow so hard, that you are trying to get about 80 percent of the air in your lungs out in the first second.*

Before you object to the accuracy of this script, let me explain why I say these words. Because people GET IT. Coaching this way produces better peak expiratory flows (PEF) and optimal FEV1s because clients/patients understand the concept of getting most of the air out of the lungs right away.

We are taught to coach the client by saying, "Blow it out as hard as you can, for as long as you can." This is a true statement, but it is sometimes difficult for people to tell just how forcibly they actually blew out. Some think they blew very hard, but the graph does not indicate it. That is why I tell them the importance of getting most of the air (around 80 percent) out in the first second. We are attempting to get a good peak flow in order to get an accurate FEV1. Although we know that some patients with severe COPD and air trapping may not expire 80 percent of the air in their lungs in the first second, the idea is presented to them in a way that they understand the *effort* that is required to obtain a good test.

Beware! Some will try to blow more slowly and pace the breath so they can blow out longer. But this strategy skews the results. They actually need to BLAST out that breath!

Many people, especially those with severe air trapping, will quit the forced exhalation before they are empty. Therefore, coach them to blow out *until* you tell them to inhale again. Of course, you will have to be watching the graph and the timer to ensure a minimum six second exhalation. After the first effort, you will be able to see if your patient has air trapping. How long do you let them exhale? Refer to Chapter Five (Coaching the COPD Group).

Lung Volume Scripts

Lung volume testing reveals total lung capacity (TLC), inspiratory capacity (IC), expiratory reserve volume (ERV), and residual volume (RV). This test will confirm restrictive lung disease (RLD) in which all the volumes are reduced, or an increase in RV found in air trapping, or an overall increase in TLC as seen in hyperinflation.

There are several testing methods:

1. Nitrogen (N2) Washout: The client performs a slow vital capacity (VC) and

then breathes 100 percent oxygen for two to seven minutes, until the N2 in the lungs is washed out, down to 1.2 percent.

2. Helium Equilibration: The client breathes 10 percent helium until equilibration is reached between the lungs and the spirometer. This usually takes two to three minutes for normal lungs and up to seven minutes for diseased lungs.

3. Body Plethysmography or Body Box: Lung volumes, Airway Resistance (RAW) and Thoracic Gas Volumes (VTG) are obtained as the client sits in the box with the door closed, performing a slow vital capacity test, then shallow, rapid panting to obtain RAW and VTG values.

Nitrogen Washout Coaching Script

A Nitrogen Washout test usually takes only a few minutes for a client with normal lungs. However, someone with air trapping in the lungs may be breathing five to seven minutes on the machine and may find it difficult.

Pre-Test Coaching:

- *For this test you will start out breathing normally.*

- *Then, I'll ask you to slowly empty out your lungs all the way until you are completely empty.*

- *Next, I'll ask you to inhale, slow and steady, all the way in until you are completely full.*

- *Then you will breathe normally for the rest of the test.*

Either an inspiratory vital capacity (IVC) or an expiratory vital capacity (EVC) is acceptable. Coach your patient during the Nitrogen Washout test using this as a guide, using the IVC method:

- *After you have the mouthpiece in your mouth and nose clips on, just breathe normally.*

- *OK, now exhale a-l-l-l the way out until you are very, very empty.*

- *Keep going, keep going.*

- *Now, inhale a-l-l-l the way in until you are very, very full. Keep going, all the way in.*

- *Great. Now, breathe normally again.*

- *Keep breathing normally for the rest of the test.*

This coaching script is a short, concise statement eliminating the need to say that the test may take five to seven minutes, since you really don't know how long it will take. Normal lungs test faster than diseased lungs. This knowledge can work against the patient who thinks, "I can't do much more of this." Instead, talk with continual encouragement, keeping your client focused on your words, and not on his/her breathing. That's right. It's a diversion and Mac Law 4 (Encourage Now, Then & Again.)

Usually, it is not necessary to tell the patient he/she would be breathing 100 percent oxygen during this test. Why? Because there will always be someone who says, "What about oxygen toxicity?" Then, I would have to encourage the client to overcome an unfounded fear.

However if the patient is on oxygen 24/7, to alleviate anxiety, I will mention that oxygen is delivered through the machine during this test. Try to evaluate each patient as you go. For example, if your patient has normal lungs and no apprehension, that patient probably would not object to breathing 100 percent oxygen for a few minutes. Some have even liked the idea!

Body Plethysmography (Body Box) Coaching

The body plethysmograph test uses a booth that has clear walls and door (to decrease claustrophobia) in which the patient sits, breathing on a mouthpiece that is attached to a pneumotach. It measures lung volumes by determining thoracic gas volume (VTG). It measures and calculates TLC, VC, FRC, ERV, RV, and RV/TLC. It also obtains RAW and sGAW values.

It is considered the most accurate method to determine lung volumes because it measures all the air in the thorax, including trapped air.

Can you really get good results without pulling you hair out? Yes, you can. Just tweak your coaching and use the following scripts as guides.

Pre-Test Coaching:

- *This is the only test that will be done with the door closed, but the test goes quickly.*

- *I'll explain the test so that you know what to expect.*

- *But you don't have to memorize anything because I will coach you as you are doing the test.*

- *You will start out with normal breathing on the mouthpiece with the nose clips on your nose.*

- *Then, I'll ask you to exhale gently all the way out until you are very, empty.*

- *Next, fill up your lungs slowly with as much air as you can—all the way in.*

(Use arm signals—this is the VC.)

- *Then, you will return to normal breathing.*

- *At the end, you will put your hands on your cheeks like this, and the only reason for that is so air won't go into your cheeks for this part of the test.*

- *At this point, I'll say, 'Pant,' and you will pant gently in and out, in and out, with small puffs of air, like this.* (Demonstrate and let the patient practice the panting maneuver.)

Hint: I have found it helpful to hold up a tissue a few inches in front of my mouth, as I demonstrate light panting. Then have the patient try it. This is an effective visual aid that helps the patient to gauge the depth of the panting efforts.

- *You'll pant for several breaths; then, at the end of the test you will feel the mouthpiece close off for the last few puffs*

(Hint: If you had the patient do the maximum inspiratory/expiratory pressure (MIP/MEP) tests already, you can mention that it feels similar.)

- *But it will only be for a few seconds, while the machine gets pressure readings.*

- *Just keep your lips tight and continue the panting motion.*

The PF machine I use requires a one minute warm up for thermal equilibration, with the patient in the box with door closed. Not all PF machines require this warm-up; but, since mine does, I also say the following:

- *Now I'll close the door and will let you know when to get on the mouthpiece.*

- *We will let the machine warm up for a little bit first.*

In keeping with Mac Law 2 (Less Info, Better Results), you do not need to warn clients that it will be a minute warm-up time, unless they ask. A minute can seem like a long time for someone suffering from claustrophobia. While waiting for the warm-up, I will turn on the box intercom and ask if they can hear me. Take your time as you talk, so the wait time goes faster for your client.

The Body Box test is considered by many as one of the most difficult of tests to perform. This is due to patient claustrophobia, inability to pant correctly, losing a mouth seal, and panicking when the shutter closes, even though warned. The best way to overcome these problems is to become a master of distraction. It is all in your coaching techniques.

Reality: I once did a PFT on an 83-year-old who couldn't do the Body Box test, but a year later did an excellent "Box" test. What changed? I did. I learned better coaching techniques.

If I said to you, "Don't think of a black flag." What would you think of? A red flag? A green flag? No, a black flag! The black flags are the negatives or difficulties of a PF test and things to avoid. Don't mention the black flags; only emphasize the positives. For example:

- *This test goes quickly; it only takes a couple of minutes.*

- *You don't have to work at the panting; just do small puffs of air in and out.*

- *You are doing great.*

- *Great efforts.*

- *The only thing you could do to make that better is…*

- During the Body Box test, I will coach the client like this:

- *OK, I will close the door and let you know when to get on the mouthpiece.*

- *We have to let it warm up a little before we start.*

- *As I am closing the door, I say, 'If you have any trouble, just let me know.'*

- *As we are waiting for the Box to warm up, I check out the intercom and ask if he/she can hear me alright. Then, I'll chit chat to pass the time.*

- *You can get on the mouthpiece now. Use the nose clips and just start breathing normally.*

- (Usually takes around four to five breaths to get a stable baseline.)

- *You are doing well.*

- *Now, exhale all the way out until you are very empty.* (Watch for an end expiratory plateau on the graph, meaning the client is truly empty.)

- *Now, inhale all the way in, until you are completely full.* (Watch for an end inspiratory plateau on the graph, meaning the client is completely full. This is your VC.)

- *Go back to normal breathing.*

- *OK, put your hands on your cheeks and pant in and out, in and out.*

- *Good. Keep panting; keep panting.*

- *You can stop and take the mouthpiece out of your mouth and relax.*

- *Good effort.*

Evaluate the results. If need be, re-coach, using different words, or practice again, correcting problem areas.

Lung Diffusion (DLCO) Coaching Scripts

Don't be a-scared little buckaroo. Anonymous

The single-breath DLCO test is an important indicator of the condition of the alveolar capillary membranes. First, the client exhales to residual volume, then inspires a mixture of diffusion gases to total lung capacity, and holds his or her breath for ten seconds. As the breath is held, the gases diffuse over the alveolar capillary membranes. Then the client exhales at a moderate rate of speed into the PF machine, which analyzes the exhaled concentration of gases. A normal DLCO value is 25 mlCO/min/mm Hg, STPD (standard temperature and pressure dry).

DLCO is usually decreased in silicosis, asbestosis, berylliosis, sarcoidosis and pulmonary fibrosis. Emphysema is the only obstructive lung disease that shows a decrease in DLCO. However, DLCO can be increased in asthma and the reasons are unknown.

It has been taught that this is one of the most difficult pulmonary tests for the patient to do, however, you can turn that around and make it one of the easiest. First of all, change your attitude about it, simplify it, and find a better coaching script, like those below. Following Mac Law 2 (Less Info, Better Results), I do *not* say, "You will be holding your breath for ten seconds." I found it is much better to say something like this:

- *On this test, you will mostly be holding your breath, but it goes quickly.*

- *You will start by breathing normally; then, I'll ask you to empty out your lungs all the way so that you can take in a deep breath quickly—all the way in.*

- *Then, you will hold your breath, relaxing your shoulders, and keeping your lips tight.*

- *Keep holding your breath until I say, 'Blow it out all the way.'*

It's funny, but at this point in the testing, seven out of ten people will say, "Do I use the nose clips?" That always baffles me, since they have worn them for every test before this!

DLCO Coaching

Coach the patient during the test, using the following as a guide.

- *OK, put the mouthpiece in your mouth, and use the nose clips.*

- *Breathe normally.*

- *Now, take a deeper breath in; now, exhale a-l-l-l the way out—all the way until you are very empty Keep going; you are almost there.*

- *Now, inhale all the way in.* (If the inhalation is too slow, coach, "A little faster, to get it in the recommended 2.5 seconds.)

- *Good. Now, hold your breath. Hold it; keep holding it. Just a little bit longer; you're almost there.*

- *Alright. Now blow it out. Push, push, push; all the way, all the way.*

- *Good effort.*

- *Take the mouthpiece out and relax.*

Make it sound easy and you will see better results. Since I began coaching this way, I have not had one objection to the breath hold. Also, during this test, if you keep your voice level without drama and excitement, the results are much better. Use

Mac Law 3 (I Relax, You Relax, We All Relax) and coach with a calm voice.

Before the improvements in pulmonary equipment, we used to ask patients to exhale until completely empty and then raise a hand to indicate they were empty, but that didn't always work. Often, the mind will say, "I'm empty," but the sensitive pneumotach on the PF machine says air is still coming out. Many people with severe air trapping will give up too soon. If I cannot tell when they are empty, due to air trapping, I may use the hand method but encourage them to exhale even more after they raise their hand. Plus, you can look at their previous FVC and slow VC results and judge accordingly. Or, try both ways of coaching to see which is better. If you do use the hand method, be sure to coach the patient very clearly, encouraging to exhale until very empty. Again, just keep it simple.

Occasionally, you may get a little lady or man with shortness of breath, who just can't seem to hold his or her breath during the lung diffusion (DLCO) test, so you may need to drop to an eight-second breath-hold. However, you will want to avoid doing this, if possible, for accuracy of testing.

The more severe the lung disease, the more difficult it is for a patient to perform a PFT. Try to make this test sound easy for the patient by explaining it very calmly. There should be no tenseness in demeanor or voice that might spill over to the patient. If you make it sound and feel easy, your client picks up on it.

Also, I think that many technologists are afraid of the DLCO test because of a lack of understanding of it, because they confuse it with lung volume, or they have been told that it is difficult to get the client to perform properly. But don't be a-scared little buckaroo. It is not difficult; just get that into your thinking and you'll relax about it.

When you understand the single-breath DLCO mechanics, you will do better. You are simply having the patient exhale way out to residual volume so that he/she can inhale a deep breath of known diffusion gases. It is then held in the lungs for 10 seconds as it diffuses quickly from the alveoli into the capillary blood system. Then, the patient blows back that breath into the pulmonary function machine. The exhalation is analyzed, yielding a DLCO or diffusion rate. It is recommended to get a minimum of two reproducible efforts, within 3 ml CO of each other, and averaged together.

MVV Coaching Script

Maximum voluntary ventilation (MVV) is the volume of air that can be inhaled and exhaled deeply and rapidly for a specified time, usually 12 seconds. The patient must be sitting down for this test due to possible dizziness caused from hyperventilation.

Pre-Test Coaching:

- *First, you will start out breathing normally.*

- *Then, you begin breathing in and out, fast and deep, like this.* (Demonstrate)

During the MVV test, use the following as a coaching guide:

- *OK, put the mouthpiece in your mouth and nose clips on your nose.*

- *You'll begin with normal breathing.*

- *Ready, now breathe FAST and DEEP, IN and OUT, in and out.*

- *Keep going; you are doing very well, so keep going, fast and deep.* (Use arm rhythm up and down; be emphatic and dramatic!)

- *Great, you can stop and take the mouthpiece out of your mouth and relax.*

- *Good effort.*

Sticking to Mac Law 2 (Less Info, Better Results), I have found it better not to tell the client that he or she would be breathing that way for 12 to 15 seconds. Most people will object saying, "If I can."

Vigorous coaching and demonstration is very important for this test. Also, let the patient practice. Many COPDers do not have a problem with the deep breathing, but the speed may be too slow. I have done MANY tests saying, "Faster, faster, faster," but the patients continue on with the same, slow speed. They are used to breathing slowly, with larger tidal volumes (VT). That is normal for many COPDers. As you work with them, do not be discouraged because the value of this test has diminished over the years. Remember, if you do administer this test, the client must be seated, due to possible lightheadedness that can occur with rapid breathing.

MIP/MEP Coaching

MIP/MEP is maximal inspiratory pressures/maximal expiratory pressures. The MIP maneuver is normal breathing followed by a maximal exhalation, then a deep and quick inspiration against a restriction to obtain a pressure reading. The MEP test is normal breathing followed by a maximal inhalation, then forcibly exhaling against a closed mouthpiece. Pressure readings are obtained from the MIP/MEP tests which reflect respiratory muscle strength.

Hint: After the FVC test, I like to administer a MEP test because the coaching is similar to the spirometry test (on my PF machine).

MEP Pre-Test Coaching (as done on my PF machine):

- *You will start out breathing normally.*

- *Then, you will take a fast, deep breath in; then, blast it out hard.*

- *Only this time, when you blow, the mouthpiece will actually be closed off.* (Smile, while your patient looks at you with wide-eyes.)

- *Then say, but you will only blow out for a few seconds, while the machine gets a quick pressure reading.*

- *This reflects your respiratory muscle strength, so give it all you got!*

Then, after your client is on the mouthpiece, say:

- *Just breathe normally.*

- *OK, now breathe in deeply!*

- ***Blow!***

- *OK. Come off the mouthpiece and relax.*

- *Good job.*

This test is very effort-dependent and may take several attempts. Vigorous coaching is necessary to obtain good results. After the first MEP effort, let the patient relax and rest for a minute or so. Even though you coached well, occasionally, someone will take the time to tell you how surprised he/she was when the machine blocked off! Often, the first test lets the client know what to expect and the efforts usually get better from there.

The pulmonary function machine I use has predicted normals for each client. However, in a normal adult, a MEP is greater than 80 cm H_2O. The MEP is decreased with neuromuscular problems, emphysema, cystic fibrosis, and chronic bronchitis.

MIP Pre-Test Coaching:

- *On this test, you will do the opposite of the last test* (MEP).

- *You start with normal breathing. Then, I will ask you to exhale completely, all the way out.*

- *Then, I will say to suck in fast and deep!*

- *It feels as though you have a very thick milkshake and a very small straw and you are trying to get that milkshake out of there!* (Demonstrate)

During the test, say something like this:

- *Just breathe normally for a while.*

- *OK. Exhale all the way out until you are very empty.*

- *Now, suck in deep!*

- *Great effort. Relax, and take the mouthpiece out of your mouth.*

MIP is decreased in neuromuscular diseases that affect respiratory muscles, the diaphragm, and in spinal deformities, myasthenia gravis, polio, tetanus, Guilliane-Barre, Muscular Dystrophy, and Multiple Sclerosis.

Chapter 5

PEOPLE GROUPS

Next, we will examine some people groups commonly seen in the pulmonary function setting. Each group is discussed and reviewed in light of the Mac Laws, showing ways to improve coaching skills and methods.

Coaching the COPD Group

COPD or chronic obstructive pulmonary disease is airway obstruction caused by emphysema, chronic bronchitis, or asthma, or a combination of the diseases. COPDers fall into a group because they have many similar characteristics when it comes to pulmonary function testing. Even though COPD affects introverts, extroverts, the nervous, the calm-spirited, and all types, they eventually fall into a category. Some drag oxygen around with them and some don't. Some are in their forties and some in their sixties, but *they all have a common problem: the inability to breathe efficiently*. It can be depressing to some and others will suffer in silence. Some never stop smoking and others are so frightened that they fully cooperate with the doctors.

Some studies have shown that COPDers exhibit high incidents of depression, anxiety, and apathy. Often, they will have a strong defensive mechanism and denial system resulting in a very controlled, emotional stance or state. You will observe some COPDers weighted down by these negative traits due to the nature of the disease.

COPDers usually do not look forward to a PFT because it can be uncomfortable and difficult to perform. Your job is to make it as pleasant as possible for them, without unnecessary pressure.

The condition of a patient's lungs is always a mystery until the first FVC is performed. You don't know if you will see normal lungs, obstruction, obstruction with air-trapping, restriction, or a combination of obstruction and restriction. Pay attention to the results of the first FVC. It will direct you toward the proper coaching method for that individual.

COPD and other obstructive lung diseases cause varying degrees of air trapping in the lungs, making exhalation difficult. A forced exhalation (FVC) requires much energy and may be very tiring. Therefore, if your client is on oxygen, be sure to allow for the use of it between tests. But take the nasal cannula off during a test, as it will alter the test results if a flow is running.

The degree of difficulty is directly related to the degree of air trapping. The worse the air trapping, the longer it takes to empty out. Some clients never do, even after 15 or 20 seconds. So, how long do you let them exhale? Some physicians prefer that patients forcibly exhale for no longer than ten seconds to avoid any adverse effects, such as discomfort, fatigue, and lightheadedness. ATS/ERS believe a forced exhalation longer than 15 seconds has little value in changing clinical decisions. They recommend a minimum of six seconds or reduced airflow to 25 ml/second as an ending of the forced expiration. Children may forcibly exhale three seconds or more. But, for adults, always get the minimum six-second forced exhalation; and, after that, watch the patient and evaluate the degree of difficulty.

If you push too hard, the efforts deteriorate quickly and your client becomes discouraged. Find the right balance. If you have a patient who is struggling in discomfort during the FVC, they may, of course, end the test at any time.

One adverse effect seems to be occurring with more frequency. That is, the patient gets close to blacking out (syncope) or does, indeed, black out at the end of the forced expiration. My own observation is that it is occurring most frequently in people who are overweight and have short necks, especially males. So, if a client fits that profile, watch closely, to avoid this problem.

As you coach your patient, don't keep your eyes glued to the computer screen. Instead, look back and forth from screen to your client. Also, watch the eyes. If you see that glazed "far away" look in the eyes, STOP the test immediately and go to the client's side to steady him or her. When you speak to the client during this episode, he or she may not be able to hear you until snapping out of it, which usually only takes a few seconds.

COPD and The Mac Laws

Let's review the universal PFT Mac Laws because you will use them from the first moment you lay eyes on your client.

Mac Law 1: Please Don't Shout—Communicate

Mac Law 2: Less Info, Better Results

Mac Law 3: I Relax, You Relax, We All Relax

Mac Law 4: Encourage Now, Then and Again

Mac Law 5: My Attitude is Everything

As you receive your client, put a smile on your face, Mac Law 4, and always introduce yourself. People want to know who you are and your job title. I see so many healthcare professionals neglect this simple ice-breaker. This communication is not only proper and courteous, it immediately introduces a relaxed atmosphere

(Mac Law 3). Start out with a positive attitude (Mac Law 5) confident you are going to get good testing performance from your client. Be compassionate and empathetic to his or her breathing struggles. Using Mac Law 3, accommodate the client by hooking him or her up to your oxygen source, whether a concentrator or piped-in oxygen, if you have it available, rather than using up the client's little oxygen bottles. Offer a tissue, water, or other things that may make the visit more comfortable. Smile and chit chat. Many clients have low self-esteem and need to feel that they are important. Treat them like they are people who matter because they do. Showing a genuine interest in your client has great rewards.

Your coaching skills are critical to success. Use Mac Law 2 and give simple instructions. The less complicated, the better. Actually, some people may not be listening to you at first because they are busy examining your clothes and jewelry, or listening to your accent, or wondering from what part of the country you came. You will know if they were distracted by the results of the first test.

Remember to use Mac Law 1 and control your voice, volume, pitch and tone. Choose words of empathy and understanding for the patients with COPD. Breathing struggles dominate their lives. Every minute is regulated by timed nebulizer treatments, and medications embrace their schedule. Some clients have a world reduced to the short leash of an oxygen hose. For them, a simple trip to the doctor's office takes planning; arranging a ride, carrying oxygen devices, getting up early to take medications, and withholding bronchodilators for four to six hours before a PFT. The life of a person with COPD is not easy, so try to make the PFT as uncomplicated as possible. Your kindness will be appreciated.

Restrictive Lung Disease (RLD) Group

Restrictive lung disease is a disease process causing inflammation of the alveolar walls and fibrotic changes, leading to stiffness and resulting in reduced lung volumes. The reductions are seen in the lung volume tests, done by body box, nitrogen washout, and helium equilibration.

Some of the diseases and conditions associated with RLD are asbestosis, silicosis, sarcoidosis, congestive heart failure, Guillain-Barre syndrome, obesity, kyphoscoliosis and medications, such as Amiodarone, Methotrexate and Bleomycin. I have a lot of sympathy for these patients because they are the least understood by technicians who administer spirometries.

Reality: For example, a gentleman told me he just hated these tests because he had to do them at his job and the technician made him so frustrated by insisting he blow out longer. He said he tried and tried and, then, finally walked out because the technician said he wasn't doing the test properly. When I tested him in our lab, I immediately noticed that he blew out ALL his air within two seconds, and then was truly empty.

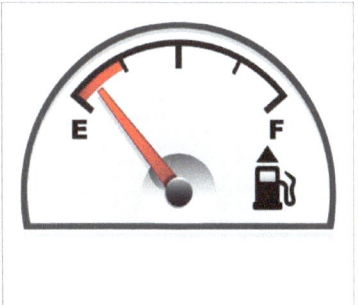

"I'm Empty!"

So how do you coach a person with RLD to push out air for six seconds when he or she is empty? Or do you have to? Actually, it is easier than you think.

First, let's look at how to coach the patient with RLD. Coaching this way has proved very successful, reducing frustration for both the patient and the technician. It has also proven to work for those with a mixture of restrictive and obstructive lung disease. And, it satisfies many physicians who consider an adequate forced exhalation to be six seconds or longer.

FVL Pre-test Coaching:

- *You'll be on the mouthpiece with the nose clips on, and I will ask you to breathe normally for just a few breaths.*

- *Next, I'll ask you to take in a deep breath—as deep as you can.*

- *Then, I'll say BLOW and just blast it out as hard as you can UNTIL I say to take another deep breath in.*

- *If you run out of air before I say to take in another deep breath, don't take a breath, but continue like you are letting the air out or even hold your breath, if you have to, and it will just be a few seconds before I ask for that last, deep breath in.*

- *Now, the most important part of this test is the first second, when I say, "Blow."*

- *You will try to get most of your air out in the first second.*

First, get a spirometry attempt:

- *Ok, put the mouthpiece in your mouth and nose clips on and breathe normally.*

- *Deep breathe in, all the way* (raising arm, pointing up).

- *Blow!* (drop arm quickly) *Keep blowing, keep blowing. It's still coming out, almost there.*

- *OK, deep breath in, fast and deep.*

- *Great effort. Relax and take the mouthpiece out of your mouth.*

Second, examine the graph. With restriction, it shows that the total volume of air is forcibly exhaled within a few seconds. That brings the forced vital capacity (FVC) value very close to the amount of air the client could blow out in the first second (the FEV1).

Third, you will not "make" your client blow out longer than necessary. Instead, coach the patient to last for six seconds by saying, *"hold your breath, if you have to,"* or *"keep pushing it out, even if you feel empty."* So often the mind says, "I'm empty," but the sensitive pneumotach is still detecting some airflow.

For spirometries, I have discovered that you may *initially* coach a person with RLD using much the same words as when coaching someone with obstructive lung disease. This is because you do not really know the condition of your client's lungs until the first FVC is done. They may have obstructive lung disease or restrictive lung disease or a mixture. If you suspect RLD, then you will coach for an expiration of six seconds but no more. If obstructive lung disease is suspected, you will coach the patient to blow out longer, such as ten to twelve seconds. The difference is that *you* control the length of time a person exhales. You'll get better results this way and most people will be able to blow out or last the full six seconds. Most people understand that they will continue to push out the air and they do so.

The "I Can't" Character

"For as he thinks in his heart, so is he"…. Proverbs 23:7

We all know this person: the negative, unhappy, arguing individual who wants to make this experience as difficult as possible for you, since he or she has to suffer through it, too. Not everyone in this world is happy, so why not just learn how to handle this personality to make it as painless as possible for you and the patient? After all, we need to get good results for the doctor, right? Keeping that in mind will help relieve any frustration you may experience. Also, here's some encouragement for you: it is important for you to realize that you CAN get good PFT tests on most of the people you test. Yes, even the "I Can't" character.

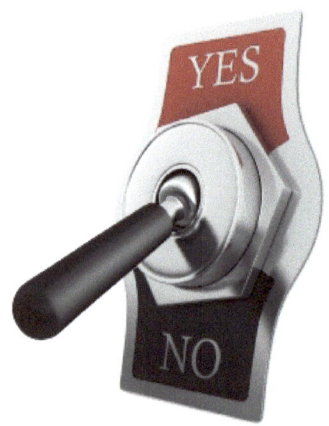

Flip the Switch

This person will say, "I can't do it," and that becomes the client's reality. Psychologists teach about self-fulfilled prophecy, in which people with negative beliefs limit themselves on what they can do. On the other hand, positive people with positive beliefs usually glide into success.

So, what possible advice can I give to the PF tech? The best way to deal with the negative person is by using Mac Law 2 (Less Info, Better Results) and give minimal instructions—just enough so they get the idea of what they will be doing. If you give them too much information, they are already thinking about how they *can't* do it, or they think they have to memorize it, or it is just too much information at one time.

Reality: A patient with restrictive lung disease came in for a PFT. He started out by saying, "I can't take in a deep breath; I can't blow out. I can't, I can't, I can't." But I knew he could do the tests because he did a PFT test the prior year, which included a pre and post bronchodilator spirometry, body plethysmography, MIP/MEP, and DLCO. I explained to him that we were just going to measure the lung capacity that he had and that he should do the best he can.

Don't give an opportunity to say "No, I can't," or any negative comment. Don't ask if they are claustrophobic. Don't put a negative thought into their head; they'll latch on to it and run with it. Then you will have to get creative in overcoming the negativity through diversion tactics.

Reality: I've heard many COPDers say, "I can't blow out long. I don't have any air." However, we know that they can because of the air trapping. But, don't argue or even try to explain about air trapping. Some just panic when they "feel" empty and then will take a deep breath or come off the mouthpiece and gasp for air. So, how do you encourage this patient?

Using Mac Law 2, never tell the "I Can't" patient how long he/she will be expected to hold that breath (for the DLCO test) or the length of time to blow out for the FVC test. Say positives only, such as, "This test takes less than a minute to do." Also, I usually do not even respond to negative comments, but still be polite and listen. Respond positively, if necessary. This kicks in Mac Law 3, (I Relax, You Relax, We All Relax).

Use Mac Law 4 and smile a lot, converse about something positive, and give lots of praise. Mac Law 5 is your challenge to self-control in administering the tests without getting frustrated.

The Impossibles

Unfortunately, there are people from whom it is impossible to get an acceptable pulmonary function test. One woman told me she couldn't do it and she proved it.

Reality: A patient in her fifties came into the PF room and just looked at the body plethysmography (body box) and said, "You're not going to shut that door are you? I'm claustrophobic. I'm not getting in there."

Immediately, I knew how to coach. I said, "OK, we can substitute a different test," thinking we could substitute the nitrogen washout for the body box. So, we started the FVC. She put the mouthpiece in her mouth, took two breaths, then suddenly grabbed her chest—like Fred Sanford in Sanford & Son—and came off the mouthpiece, gasping. Even through all the drama, her pulse oximetry showed a normal oxygen saturation of 92 percent, and heart rate of 74 beats per minute.

When questioned about what she was experiencing, she said she just gets "spasms." She agreed to try more testing but would quit prematurely and come off the mouthpiece in a panic. The only results I obtained from her were one FVC and one DLCO. Consequently, I submitted the results to the physician for his review, noting the client's panic. I made it clear, however, that acceptable and repeatable tests, according to ATS/ERS standards, were not achieved. Unfortunately, this woman was unable to control her panic, but I gave her credit for trying.

The Teen Phenomenon

Yes, teenagers have earned their own category. They are a special breed in the pulmonary function lab and they seem to interpret words differently from adults. Perhaps it is because they are in the precarious place between puberty and adulthood. Whatever the reason, you may get very exasperated in attempting just a simple spirometry (FVC) test on a teenager or young adult.

It seems to begin at approximately age 12 to about 20 years of age. What am I talking about, you ask? Obviously you never attempted a PFT on a teen. This is what happens: I'll coach the individual to "Blast it out hard!" The teen will sigh. Yes, sigh, and a slow sigh at that!

I have seen this over and over. Hmmmmm….The adult says, "Blast it out hard and the teen thinks "big sigh." Now, your challenge begins. Your communication skills must be in high gear. Since an FVC is an effort-dependent test, your coaching skills will now be tested to the limit.

Reality: I asked a pediatrician if this was my imagination or had she experienced this situation, as well. She said, "Yes, I know what you mean. It is a phenomenon."

Reality: "GI Asthma Joe" We did PFTs for military entrance candidates. The young men and women who came in required FVC testing for determination of asthma. A well-done FVC, before and after bronchodilation was required for entrance into the military, if there was a previous history of asthma or breathing disorders. Therefore, it was vitally important to get acceptable and reproducible tests. If not, their whole future and career could be altered. Yet, we saw it over and over again…sigh, not blow.

OK, that means we need to find ways to get good PFTs on these people. Believe me, I've tried everything and do have some suggestions.

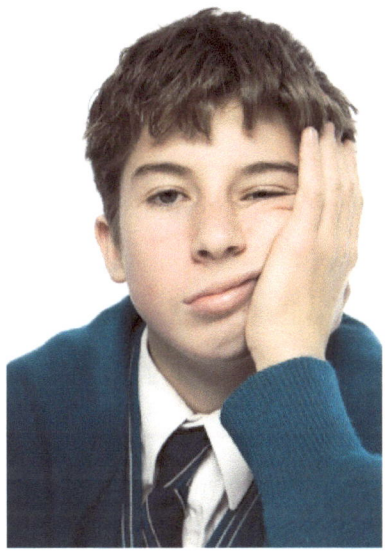

The Teen Phenomenon

1. You know that disinterested, bored attitude some teens have? It seems to reflect in their body language, as well. Getting them to sit up straight and not slouch will be your first victory. Many times, I'll just have them stand to do a FVC. But, when they blow, don't let them hunch over at the waist.

2. Demonstrate, demonstrate. Show each step, and demonstrate how to blow out forcibly.

3. When you say "BLOW," raise your voice a notch or two. It seems to work better, possibly because elevated sound levels are what they're used to hearing.

4. If you have to, do the maximum eight attempts. But don't overdo it. After a failed attempt, say, "What you could do to make that better is"….

5. Draw a picture of a normal flow volume loop and compare it to the flattened loop your client is producing. Then use Mac Law 2 (Less Info, Better Results) and briefly explain, "What you can do to improve this is to blow out much harder and faster, especially on that first second, when I say BLOW. You are actually trying to blow out 80 percent or more of your air in the first second."

6. Sometimes, it is difficult to determine if a patient is truly blasting out that first second of air as forcibly as possible, but the Peak Flow will tell you if it is an optimal effort. Be sure to get a maximal inspiration first, to get a better peak flow, which is considered the highest flowrate of the curve.

7. Tell your client that the forced exhalation cannot be paced over time.

8. Again, use Mac Law 2 (Less Info, Better Results) and do not tell them how

many seconds they will be blowing out.

9. Use Mac's Law 3 (I Relax, You Relax, We All Relax). You may think the teen is too relaxed, as seen in the slouchy body position; however, what you see is probably more indifference than anything else. The calm, cool indifference covers the uneasiness and apprehension of passing a test for which this teen patient didn't study. Engage the teen in conversation about school, future careers, talents, sports, music and anything else that may be calming. Have him/her do relaxed breathing techniques such as diaphragmatic breathing or even pursed-lip breathing, which have an overall, calming effect.

10. Use Mac Law 4 (Encourage Now, Then, & Again). Positive and encouraging words will lighten the atmosphere. Choose your words carefully so that your client doesn't feel your criticism or his or her failure.

11. Use Mac Law 5 (Your Attitude is Everything). Normally, early adolescents aged 12 to 14 years old, struggle with a sense of identity. Middle Adolescence (14 – 17 years) is more of a fragile time because they are wavering between dependence on parents and thinking independently. Their high expectations of people and situations are unrealistic and they still suffer from a poor self-image in the struggle to find identity. Finally, in Late Adolescence (17 – 19 years), there occurs more of a break toward independence as the self-image, identity, and emotions become more stable. Understanding the struggles of the adolescent may assist you in restructuring your dialog and coaching techniques. Because the teen's identity is still unsure, you will be the mentor, showing the teen how an adult acts.

12. Occasionally, if your adolescent is young enough and not in the

independent-thinking stage, it may help to get Mom or Dad in the room.

Ah, sweet success. Your patient has accomplished acceptable FVC values, but the results fall into the borderline of normal range. Would you give this patient a bronchodilator medicine?

Let's follow a critical thinking path:

- The adolescent is having this test due to some complaint of shortness of breath or similar breathing problems. So, you will be administering a PFT test to determine if airflow limitations exist.

- A PFT is to the lungs as an EKG is to the heart. Both can diagnose problems.

- Oftentimes, it is a reactive airway problem or asthma.

- We know that asthma is an inflammatory, obstructive lung disease of the small airways, which favorably responds to a bronchodilator drug.

- The degree of reversibility (how much the airways open up) after the administration of a bronchodilator, such as Albuterol, is significant in diagnosing asthma. Even a borderline-normal FEV1 may dramatically open up the airways after bronchodilation.

- You decide to administer a bronchodilator. A metered-dose inhaler (MDI) is the preferred choice for PF testing. Some labs give nebulizer treatments.

- You wait the appropriate length of time, which is 15 minutes for a short-acting Beta 2-agonist bronchodilator.

- The patient produces three more acceptable post-bronchodilator spirometries. But, this time, it will be easier, since your teen has mastered the testing procedure.

The results are in, but what do they mean? There is no absolute agreement as to what earmarks a good response to a bronchodilator due to a variety of factors. Some consider a 12 percent or greater increase in FEV1 and/or FVC, to be significant. Consult with your medical director for his/her recommendations.

I have often wondered if there is a physiological reason for the Teen Phenomenon. Maybe someone will do a study on it someday! Anyway, what I recommend is to try your best, and follow the Mac Laws. If you are submitting the client's best efforts, be sure to chart accordingly. If substandard results are submitted, clearly chart any deviations or problems. You may chart whether, in your opinion, the test results were acceptable.

Why is it important to be clear in your charting? You will chart enough information so that the physician looking at the test doesn't think that the teen has an upper airway obstruction and order a bronchoscopy. We know that a poor inspiration on a spirometry graph can look like an extrathoracic obstruction. A poorly forced expiratory effort produces a flattened expiratory graph, which looks like an intrathoracic obstruction.

Hint: If a coaching attempt fails, you must change up your coaching words or technique. Try a better explanation or a different script. Don't get discouraged. It's not you, it's the Teen Phenomenon.

The Controller

Ah, the "Type A" person who doesn't wait for you to finish your explanation, saying, "I know, I know." They are on the mouthpiece huffing and puffing before they know what to do!

They are more comfortable controlling their environment and usually do not like to be told what to do. You will find that many patients with breathing problems are anxious and the Controller is no exception. By coaching them tactfully, you help them to relax, so they can listen better and perform the tests properly. If you follow these suggestions, just watch and see their fears subside.

After you have detected a Controller personality, (which should take only a few minutes of listening to the patient), you'll find it helpful to make changes in your dialog and coaching techniques.

1. Let him/her control some things. Like what? There are times you can let the client have some control, though limited, over the performance of the test. For example, on a DLCO, right before the breath-hold, I will say, "You'll breathe normally and *when you are ready, begin to exhale out,"* then take over from there and coach him/her to exhale completely. Just this small amount of control can sometimes make all the difference.

   Reality: I went a step further on an older gentleman I recently had in the PF lab. He did much better on a DLCO, when I let him determine when to inhale deeply and then exhale completely. Then, I jumped in and coached him to continue exhaling. The point is, when I let him initiate the maneuver, he was much more comfortable, cooperative and coachable.

   Reality: Another example was a young lady with cystic fibrosis who did much better on her FVC's when I let her take the first maximal breath to capacity (she knew her full capacity better than I could determine on the graph). Then, she forcefully blew out until I said, "Now, deep breath in." She had been doing FVC's since she was seven years old, so she knew the procedure well and did much better when allowed to control part of the test.

2. During your initial instruction of a test, ask, don't tell. For example: On an FVC, say, "I'll *ask* you to take a deep breath, then blast it out hard." Just one word, ask, not tell, seems to comfort the controller. Or you can say, "I'll *say* take a deep breath in...*" This is Mac Law 4 (Encourage Now, Then & Again), which works for the Controller and the majority of the general public.

3. Use Mac Law 4 and smile a lot. It is a good stress reducer because people will usually smile back and relax more. Try it; it works.

4. Be patient. Mac Law 5 (My Attitude is Everything). Understand that you can make it worse or better for your clients, depending on your attitude. Don't react by becoming a Controller yourself. It will cause the Controller to resist more.

Jittery Janet

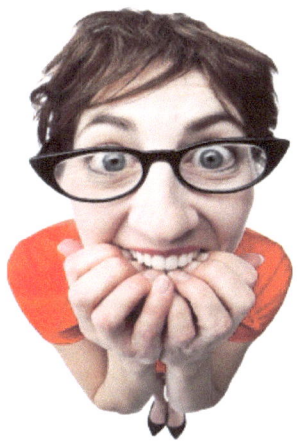

Reality: Jittery Janet came in for a test. Even though I asked her to be seated in the red chair, she just bounced around the room for a while and then said, "Do you want me to sit in the box yet?"

Immediately I realized several things about Janet:

- She didn't listen well and often said, "You didn't tell me that."

- She was trying too hard.

- She was trying to remember everything.

- She was impatient, saying, "Are we done yet?" "Another test?"

She needed from me:

- Calm reassurance.

- Humor, lots of it.

- Patience and lots of it.

All the laws go into effect for Janet. Let's apply each one.

Mac Law 1 - Please Don't Shout: Jittery people get even more nervous if we talk too loud. It is a linear relationship. Use your most calm, soothing voice with a low tone to help Jittery Janet become more comfortable with you.

Mac Law 2 - Less Info, Better Results: When you give instructions, Janet is thinking, "Oh, I can't remember all this," so reassure her that you will be coaching throughout the testing and she doesn't have to memorize anything. Use a little humor and tell her, "Don't worry; I'll be coaching you through each test as you're doing it. I'm good at telling people what to do." (Smile)

Mac Law 3 - I Relax, You Relax, We All Relax: Before testing, let Jittery Janet talk for a while. Listen for a topic that she enjoys talking about, preferably one that doesn't have anything to do with breathing. Watch how she relaxes when you get her to talk about something she likes.

Mac Law 4 - Encourage Now, Then, and Again: Smile, offer words of encouragement, and let her know that it's not a pass/fail kind of test. You'll just be measuring what she can do. Jittery Janets can experience test anxiety and try very hard to get it right. Be patient; you may have to explain things more than one time.

Mac Law 5 - Your Attitude is Everything: Finally, you must maintain a calm posture. Anything else would be disaster. You will have to put on an extra measure of patience for Janet. Just stay in control of yourself and the PFT experience.

Chapter 6

"I ONLY DO SPIROMETRIES"

OK, let's go over what you need to know to get great tests. ATS/ERS has defined what makes an FVC acceptable and repeatable. I encourage you to read their "Standardisation of Spirometry" statement online at http://www.thoracic.org/statements/resources/pfet/PFT2.pdf. You will learn what makes an acceptable FVC effort, what artifacts to watch for, what makes a good start and exhalation, and the requirements for repeatability. Also, go to http://www.cdc.gov/niosh/docs/2011-135/pdfs/2011-135.pdf and review the NIOSH spirometry chart designed to get great FVCs every time. It is an excellent chart and free to print!

Always start with a calibrated machine. This is not a suggestion, but a necessity. Turn on the machine, let it warm up the required time (check your manual), then calibrate the pneumotach with a three-liter syringe. If you do a flow/volume loop or a MVV, you must calibrate both inspiration and expiration.

Normal Norman

Let's say you give annual employee PFTs, which is just an FVC, at your workplace and most of your employees have normal lungs. This should be easy, right? I've given hundreds of them, and have found that people interpret instructions very differently. Remember the Mac Laws as you give an explanation of the FVC. I have listed several scripts here in case your client does not understand the test procedure.

If one script doesn't work, try another. Remember to use body signals, such as putting your arm all the way up for inhalation and dropping it down sharply for the forced exhalation. I've been called a cheerleader by many clients!

You will find that pulmonary function machines vary in testing methods. The FVC is usually just a deep breath in, then a forcible and prolonged exhalation, but one machine may have the client start with the mouthpiece in his/her mouth and breathing normally. Another machine may have the employee inhale completely first, *then* put the mouthpiece in and blow hard. Or, a third method is to put the mouthpiece in, take a deep breath, then blow hard. Get familiar with your own equipment and practice on yourself and others.

Prepare the patient for an FVC using the following script as a guide. Include a demonstration of the deep, quick inhalation and the forced blast out:

- *On this test, I will say, 'Take in a deep breath—all the way in.'*

- *Next, you will BLAST it out as hard and fast as you can and keep pushing it out until you are very, very empty.*

- *I will encourage you to continue to try pushing it out, by saying, 'keep going, keep going, blow, blow, blow.'*

- *Even if you feel empty, continue to blow it out or even hold it there if you have to UNTIL I say, 'Stop and relax.'*

During the FVC test, use this as a guide:

- *Please sit (or stand) up straight and put the mouthpiece in your mouth Put on the nose clips.*

- *Now put the mouthpiece in your mouth and take in a deep breath, all the way!*

- *Now BLAST it out, keep going, keep going, blow, blow, blow.*

- *Stop and relax. Remove the mouthpiece and nose clips.*

- *Very good effort.*

- *When you feel ready, we'll get another.*

Some PF machines do flow-volume loops (slang: FLOOPS), which is an FVC with a fast, maximal deep breath added to the end of the test after the forced exhalation.

For a flow-volume loop (FVL), prepare the patient using the following script as a guide:

- *You'll be on the mouthpiece, with the nose clips on, breathing normally.*

- *Then, I'll ask you to take in a deep breath—all the way in.*

- *Then, I'll say to BLAST it out hard and fast.*

- *You will blow it out as HARD as you can for as LONG as you can, or maybe a little longer!* (Smile)

- *You'll be very empty; and then, at the end, I'll ask you to take in another quick, deep breath.*

During the FVL test, enthusiastically coach:

- *OK, put the mouthpiece in your mouth, and the nose clips on your nose.*

- *Breathe normally.* (Watch to see when the patient is inhaling or exhaling.)

- *Now, take a deep breath in a-l-l-l the way.* (arm up)

- *BLOW.* (Drop arm quickly.) *Blow. Keep blowing, keep blowing. Let it out;*

push, push.

- *Almost there.*

- *Now a quick, deep breath in; all the way in.*

- *OK. Very good. You can relax now.*

It is general knowledge that a minimum exhalation of six seconds is recommended. I usually let them go longer, if they can, but no longer than 15 seconds. Be aware of the person with restrictive lung disease who is empty after only a couple seconds. Review Chapter 5, Coaching the RLD Group. If the person with RLD gives up the forced exhalation right away, you'll need to get him or her to either blow out longer or watch for a plateau. I have adapted the script to say, "Some people empty out right away; and, if you do, don't stop blowing out. Keep trying, and even hold it there if you have to, UNTIL I say to stop."

I have found that when I emphasize UNTIL, most people get it and continue blowing out. Of course, if you coach this way, you have to watch the timer to ensure an exhalation time greater than six seconds. In all the years I've coached this way, only one man didn't understand and actually closed his glottis. To avoid this situation, you can add:

Just let the air out; don't shut down the back of your throat off as you blow. Let the air continue to come out. You are controlling it.

Also, I like to coach to "blow out a little longer than you can," because so often people "feel" empty, but actually they are not. The pneumotach that measures the airflow is very sensitive in detecting whether a patient is empty or not. Also, watch your graph. Is it flattening (plateau)? Then the patient is getting empty.

If employees/clients sit for the test, both feet need to be flat on the floor, no legs crossed, and the torso upright and straight. If they stand for the test, do not let them hunch over at the waist while they forcibly blow.

The most common errors:

1. Employee posture.

2. Employee doesn't blast out hard enough.

3. Employee tries to pace the exhalation by blowing out slowly.

4. Employee is strictly a nose-breather and nose clips are not available.

5. Employee stops too soon (when he "feels" empty).

6. Lack of enthusiastic coaching by technician.

7. Technician is not clear on what makes a good FVC test. (Such as looking at the peak flow to see if the effort was good.)

8. Technician is not clear on how to change coaching script to get better results. Saying the same thing over and over to the employee may not change the results.

9. A less than maximal inhalation, resulting in variable tests.

Note on Peak Expiratory Flow (PEF):

The peak expiratory flow (also expressed as FEF max) is the maximum and highest flow achieved during the forced expiration maneuver. It reveals the patient's cooperation and effort. For example, a peak expiratory flow value less than 70 percent, that may indicate a poor expiratory effort, and the patient needs to blast it out harder. If the peak flow is less than desired, make sure the patient is getting a *maximal* inhalation before the vigorous *BLAST* out.

Next, continue reading Chapter 7 for more tips on positioning, glottis closure, mouthpieces, cleanliness, gaggers and droolers, and more Real-Life experiences.

Chapter 7

TIPS, TRICKS AND TECHNIQUES

Keep It Clean

Germaphobe Jerrys are on the rise, and understandably so. Methicillin-resistant Staphylococcus Aureous (MRSA) is getting more prominent in the news, as new cases are being reported. MRSA can be Hospital-Acquired (HA) or Community-Acquired (CA). The Centers for Disease Control and Prevention website (http://www.cdc.gov/mrsa/) has an abundance of information about MRSA symptoms, prevention in hospitals and schools, treatment and cleanliness.

Cleanliness and good hand-washing technique is essential. Let your client see you wash your hands. Wait until the patient is ready to start the PF testing before removing the mouthpiece and filter from its package. Then, use the plastic bag, or gloves to put the mouthpiece on the machine. Never use bare hands or handle the part of the mouthpiece that goes into the client's mouth. If you drop the nose clips, replace them. Never reuse a disposable, cardboard mouthpiece!

Reality: I opened a sealed package to remove the mouthpiece, which was sealed in another plastic package. Even though the patient watched me do this, he still asked, "Is that a clean one?"

Reality: I was doing a PFT on a patient; and, between trials, a fly decided to land on the expiratory side of the pneumotach and I couldn't get him off! I waved the pneumotach back and forth, but he was stuck there. As a result, I had to change out the pneumotach and recalibrate before continuing.

Mouthpieces

There is a variety of mouthpieces for pulmonary function testing. There are cardboard mouthpieces for the small spirometry machines and large, rubber mouthpieces for gas tests, such as helium equilibration, nitrogen washout, and lung diffusion. It is highly recommended to use the rubber mouthpieces for gas tests, so there are no leaks during the test.

Another important tip is to make sure the patient has the mouthpiece in his or her mouth properly. If the teeth are not in the right position, you may get leaks. A leak means an inaccurate test; or, if the teeth are not in the correct position and your client bites down too hard, you will have an obstruction to the airflow, which, again, can alter results.

Often, I have to ask the patient to, "Put your lips forward, like you are kissing," to close the gap at the corners of the mouth, and avoid leaks.

For cardboard mouthpieces, make sure the end goes into the mouth and not up against the lips or teeth, so airflow is not obstructed. Also, ask the patient to keep the tongue out of the hole.

Reality: After many attempts at a spirometry test, my patient just couldn't seem to get an acceptable result. Everything looked right. The patient was on the mouthpiece correctly and performed the test correctly, but the graph was showing a blockage. Finally, I asked if her tongue was getting in the mouthpiece as she blew. It was then that she turned to me and stuck out her tongue. Let's just say Gene

Simmons has nothing on her! Now that I knew the problem, it was an easy fix. She put her tongue under the mouthpiece blew again and produced excellent results.

Glottis Closure

Glottis closure occurs when a person forcibly blows out for a few seconds, but then closes the glottis, which stops any more air from being exhaled. It's also called a Valsalva maneuver. Glottis closure is not common, but it does happen.

Reality: A client blew out hard for a couple seconds and then unwittingly closed his glottis. On the graph, I saw air come out for a few seconds forming a curve, then an abrupt flat line. He kept saying, "It just stops coming out." True, but he didn't realize he was doing it to himself. He was straining so hard that his face turned red and neck veins bulged.

I explained that he was straining so hard that his throat was closing up, stopping the air from coming out. To remedy this problem, I asked him to blow forcibly the first second, but then to back off somewhat as he *let* the air continue to come out. This re-coaching was sufficient to obtain good results. Again, if your client does not understand your explanation, change it until he does understand. If you say the same thing over and over, he obviously didn't get it the first time, so you need to find the right words for it to make sense to him.

What's so important about the slow Vital Capacity (VC) test?

A valid VC is important because the values are used to calculate RV (residual volume) and TLC (total lung capacity). RV and TLC reflect the degree of air trapping and hyperinflation. There are two methods, IVC (inspiratory vital capacity) and EVC (expiratory vital capacity).

During the IVC test, the client will breathe normally, in a relaxed manner, for at least three breaths until a stable baseline is achieved, then exhales completely, and finally inhales maximally to TLC. An EVC is normal, relaxed tidal breathing, then full inhalation to TLC, followed by a slow and steady exhalation to RV. It is best to have your patient use nose clips during this test.

The most common error I have observed in coaching a slow VC, is that the technician quits too early and does not coach the patient into a MAXIMAL inhalation and MAXIMAL exhalation. Coach until you see a one second plateau on the graph, which indicates your client is very full (or empty), then you know the effort was the client's best.

However, please realize that the COPDer, or emphysemic with air trapping may never empty out during an exhalation; but, the more you can get, the better for a valid RV. It may make your patient uncomfortable. Use your best clinical judgment and compare with the prior FVCs. A person with air trapping may have a higher slow VC value than FVC value.

Word Twisters

Try to speak clearly and plainly to people to avoid misunderstandings. Sometimes, words can get twisted and they hear only what they want to hear, not what you mean.

Reality: A patient with severe, end-stage COPD came in for a test. A few days later his pulmonologist asked me why I told this patient he had good lungs. Of course, I hadn't. As we discussed my coaching methods, it seemed that when I encouraged the patient saying, "good job, good effort," he interpreted it as, "my lungs are good!" Perhaps he was in denial, but this example illustrates how careful we should be in choosing our words. Ever since that experience, I make it clear to the patient that I am only evaluating his efforts, not the results.

Giver-Uppers

This is the patient who blows out for one to two seconds on the forced exhalation on the FVC maneuver, then gives up and stops or takes in a breath before the six second minimum is achieved. Try this:

When you say to blow, say it like this: "Blooooooooowwwwwwwww," until they pass the six second mark. Be sure to take in a deep breath yourself, so you can make your "Blooooooooowwwwwwwww" last. This strategy works very well. People just seem to stay in tune with you and continue the exhalation as long as you are saying, "Blooooooooooooooooooowwwwwww."

Gaggers and Droolers

Mr. Gagger, true to form, put the mouthpiece in his mouth, blew a little, then started gagging. Being one myself, I understand that it is a natural problem, but most people seem to be able to overcome it as they continue the testing. Just have plenty of tissue handy.

The Dreaded Nose Clips!

Unfortunately, many people have an aversion to wearing nose clips for pulmonary function testing.

Reality: A lady came in for a test one day and I put the nose clips on her. She literally quit breathing! Finally, she grabbed the clips and threw them, gasping for air! She was not able to perform a PFT at all.

Reality: A woman was claustrophobic; and, when nose clips were placed on her nose, she'd do OK for a few breaths, then panic. I managed to get only one acceptable FVC. She tried several DLCO's and a N2 Washout, but without success.

Remedy: Most people can retrain themselves to breathe only through the mouth. Some people will do better if you let them hold their own noses and chunk the nose clips. Giving the patient some control seems to work better. Remember that many people with breathing issues exhibit anxiety if they think they can't breathe.

Test Accuracy

- When doing repeat PFTs, be sure to check that the "predicted norms" are the same as the last test.

- Always check the height and weight of the patients for accuracy. Sometimes, if you ask, "How tall are you?" They'll say, "Well, my driver's license says..." Let the tape measure be the final authority. Measure and chart that you did the check.

- Insert the correct race for the accurate, predicted norms. Why is this important? People of some races have smaller lungs and there is a correction factor for that.

- If you get a client with supra-normal values, always double-check that you entered the birth date height and weight correctly.

- Other important details: The PF machine has been calibrated prior to patient testing, and all calibrations are logged and up to date. If you have more than one co-worker, double-check each other's tests. Also, it is recommended that a pulmonary lab have a Biological Control, where one or two people with normal lungs perform a complete PF test every month, or as often as required by the medical director. Each test is compared to the last and observed for changes.

Positioning

Ask the patient to sit up with back straight and mouth level with the mouthpiece. Make adjustments as needed. Both feet need to be flat on the floor and about a shoulder width apart. Arms need to be down at the sides, not crossed in front of the chest, which could restrict breathing. It is recommended for pediatric patients to stand up for the FVC test and do not let them hunch over when blowing out.

Reality: Some physicians want all adult PFTs done with the patient standing. If you do this, do not let the patient stand for the MVV (maximum voluntary ventilation) test because, after breathing deeply at a rate of >70 bpm for 15 seconds, you may have your arms full, as he or she may not be standing by the end of the test.

Reality: A patient came in for a PFT. As I was coaching him in the first FVC, about 5 seconds into the forced exhalation, he suddenly had a glazed look in his eyes and quit responding to me. I quickly went over to his side to steady him. He came very close to passing out.

This is what I learned from this incident and others to follow: Some people, especially those with a short, thick neck and overweight, have a tendency to pass out or get close to syncope at the end of the FVC expiratory maneuver. I would not advise letting him/her stand up for the PFT. It seems that in our overweight society, we are seeing with more frequency the patient who exerts so much "push" on the spirometry that, at the very end of the forced exhalation, the patient passes out. Watch the eyes for that "far-away" look; and, if you see it, STOP THE TEST IMMEDIATELY.

If the test has gone too far, these patients will not hear your commands to stop, so get ready to catch them if you have to do so. I have seen people completely pass out or get close to passing out. ATS explains the syncope occurs from an extended interruption of venous return to the thorax. If you keep a careful watch on their eyes, and do not let them exhale excessively long, you can hinder it from happening. I trained employees to look at the patient, then to look at the computer screen, back and forth, so as to protect the patient.

Troubleshooting

I've worked with a wide variety of pulmonary function machines such as Viasys, MedGraphics, Collins, Sensormedics, and even the Gould machine, back in the 1980's. When it comes to troubleshooting, each has its own little quirks. You will get used to the machine you work with and will recognize when a balloon bursts and learn how to change it. Watch for changes from "normal." Learn to recognize mouthpiece "leaks" by watching the patient and observing the graph as it keeps dropping. Lastly, listen to your "gut" feeling. It usually steers you in the right direction.

Cough It Up!

Reality: A patient with severe COPD had a decreased, post-bronchodilator FVC and FEF25-75%. After coughing up secretions, his FEF25-75% improved.

Overweight and Embarrassed

Many patients preparing for bariatric surgery are embarrassed to answer the question, "How much do you weigh?" So, as soon as they answer, I quickly ask them, "Have you ever smoked?" This little diversion helps lessen the embarrassment and a little kindness goes a long way.

Disability Dan

Reality: We did all the disability PFTs and one day a man came in just huffing and puffing, saying, "I can't breathe, I can't breathe." He really put on a show and his FVC attempts were pitiful. He wanted to prove to me how bad his lungs were. I finally had to tell him that all his attempts were not acceptable per disability standards and his claim would probably be denied. He was astounded! I then explained that we are just trying to measure what he could do, but I needed his cooperation in performing the tests in the proper manner. Suddenly, he began to blast out his air forcibly, proving he had normal lungs.

Reality: Another man showed up intoxicated at 9:30 AM. I informed him that he needed to be sober to perform the tests properly so he had to reschedule.

Reality: Still another client came in coughing and then, when asked to Blow,

Blow, Blow, he exhaled slowly. Again, I re-coached saying, "This machine can tell if you are blowing out as hard as you can. I know you can because I see that your cough is strong and forceful. You don't want to be disqualified by disability, so please blast it out harder." He cooperated after that.

Wheelchairs

Wheelchairs may present another challenge. Don't give up; be inventive. Patients may need a pre-op PFT for surgery. If they are wheelchair-bound, your method of testing for lung volumes may have to be a helium dilution or nitrogen washout. If they can get into the body box, that would be your first choice.

Smokin' Sam—"I'll smoke 'til I die!"

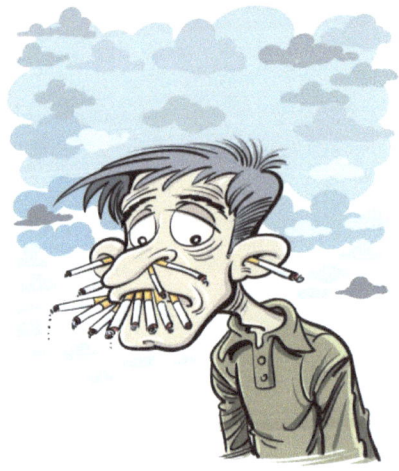

Smokin' Sam

Reality: A client was sitting in the PF lab, getting oxygen through his nasal cannula and he defiantly informed me "I'll smoke 'til I die!" Previously, at his doctor's insistence, he tried to quit, but complained that the medication to help him stop smoking was just too expensive. Then, he said his wife smokes, too. I added up the cost of cigarettes for this family of two, and, at that time, it was about $345.00 a month. The medication was not as expensive as the cigarettes, but the plain fact was that he just didn't want to quit. Smokers have increased hospital stays, bronchitis, medication usage, and arterial and lung damage. The physician taking care of Smokin' Sam said to me, "Did you get him to quit smoking? I've been trying for 10 years!"

Frisky Frank/Frisky Francine

If you have a client in your lab that seems a little too frisky for your liking, keep the door open or ask another PF technician to take over, who is the same sex as your client.

Reality: My male co-worker always seemed to know when Frisky Frank was at the PF machine and would take over for me, saving me from off-colored comments and jokes.

Pre- and Post-Bronchodilator Spirometry

Bronchodilation is recommended if FVC, FEV1 and FEF25-75% are reduced and for a determination of asthma. Albuterol or Xopenex via metered-dose inhaler (MDI) or nebulizer may be given for bronchodilation. The MDI is the preferred method for PFTs, however, this may be determined by the Medical Director or by an approved PFT protocol. An MDI is a small, handheld inhaler which delivers one puff or dose, of medicine at a time.

If you give an MDI for bronchodilation, use a spacer with a one-way valve in it, called a valved holding chamber. This is a device used with some metered dose inhalers to deliver a more effective dosage into the lungs. Examples vary from plastic tubes to cardboard pop-ups.

Have the patient exhale completely, then inhale maximally (but not quickly because the medication will go deeper if the air is not turbulent.) Then, the patient will do a ten-second breath-hold as you countdown: 10-9-8-7-6-5-4-3-2-1. Wait a minute before giving the next puff in order to give the airways time to begin bronchodilation, so the next puff will go deeper.

Filter Dead Space

Filters used on pulmonary function machines have volume, such as 15 ml or 22 ml, which should be entered into the machine to correct for the volume. This is particularly important if you test children, since their own tidal volumes are small. If you do not know the volume of the filter, you can fill it with water and then measure how much water it took to fill it.

What's a PFT Protocol?

A pulmonary function test protocol is a set of guidelines which aides a PF technologist in obtaining PFTs by following an algorithm, which ensures all the necessary tests will be done. For example, if the FVC test indicates possible restrictive lung disease, following a PFT protocol will lead the technologist to administer a lung volume test, too.

How many attempts?

In order to get repeatable efforts, the following is generally accepted, but recommendations may be determined by the medical director or supervisor of the lab.

FVC: 3 to 12

DLCO: 2 to 5

MVV: 2 minimum

MIP/MEP: 2 minimum

VC: 3 to 4

I hope you find these tips helpful and now it's up to you to put them to work! Great success to you.

References

ATS/ERS Resources: http://www.thoracic.org/statements/

DelCampo, Diana S. "Understanding Teens." Bringing Science to Your Life. New Mexico State University. 1 Oct 2011. http://aces.nmsu.edu/pubs/_f/f-122.pdf

GOLD Resources: http://www.goldcopd.org/

NIOSH Resources: http://www.cdc.gov/niosh/topics/spirometry/training.html

Stage, Kurt B., et al. " Depression in COPD: management and quality of life considerations." International Journal of COPD, v. 1 (3), 2006. 315-320. <http://www.ncbi.nlm.nih.gov/pmc/articles/PMC2707161/>

About the Author

Rosemary (R.K.) McWilliams, BAS, RRT, CPFT, began her career in respiratory therapy in 1978. She says, "I started in respiratory before it was mandatory to wear gloves to draw blood! Can you imagine?" It was back in the days of glass syringes, lubed with liquid heparin, for drawing blood gases, metal tracheal tubes, and the MA-1 ventilator.

In 1986, her work led her into a specialized area of respiratory therapy—pulmonary function testing. It was an instant attraction and she knew she found her niche. It was then that Rosemary decided, as a Registered Respiratory Therapist (RRT), to add the Certified Pulmonary Function Technologist (CPFT) credential to her resume. Eventually, she went on to obtain a B.A.S. degree, with honors, from Wayland Baptist University.

As a therapist for over 35 years, she has held positions as a director of respiratory care, coordinator of a pulmonary function lab at a major hospital, worked for a pulmonologist, and at a cardiology group doing PFTs, sleep studies, and other educational training.

After many years of administering pulmonary function tests, Rosemary learned techniques and methods to make the testing procedure easier for patients and technicians. In *Airtight Pulmonary Function Testing*, she's passing on these tips, learned from real life experiences. Her desire is to make your job easier and patients receive better tests. Therefore, Rosemary is sharing this knowledge and encouragement to every life that comes in contact with a pulmonary function test.

Rosemary, has also written science fiction books under the pen name, R.K. McWilliams. Her latest novels are *Chemical Chaos, Book One of the Blood Moon Series,* available on Amazon in ebook and print, with Book Two, *Sword of Caleb,* soon to be published.

Contacts:

http://rkmcwilliams.com

Email: rk@rkmcwilliams.com

Facebook: https://www.facebook.com/AirtightPulmonaryFunctionTests

Or: https://www.facebook.com/rkmcwilliamsauthor

Twitter: rkmcwilliams@chemchaos

www.ingramcontent.com/pod-product-compliance
Lightning Source LLC
Chambersburg PA
CBHW050728180526
45159CB00003B/1159